MAN *and* WOUND
in the ANCIENT
WORLD

OTHER BOOKS BY RICHARD A. GABRIEL

Hannibal: The Military Biography of Rome's Greatest Enemy
Philip II of Macedonia: Greater than Alexander
Thutmose III: The Military Biography of Egypt's Greatest Warrior King
Scipio Africanus: Rome's Greatest General
The Battle Atlas of Ancient Military History
The Warrior's Way: A Treatise on Military Ethics
Muhammad: Islam's First Great General
Soldiers' Lives Through History
Jesus the Egyptian: The Origins of Christianity and the Psychology of Christ
Empires at War: A Chronological Encyclopedia
Subotai the Valiant: Genghis Khan's Greatest General
The Military History of Ancient Israel
The Great Armies of Antiquity
Sebastian's Cross
Gods of Our Fathers: The Memory of Egypt in Judaism and Christianity
Warrior Pharaoh: A Chronicle of the Life and Deeds of Thutmose III,
    Great Lion of Egypt, Told in His Own Words to Thaneni the Scribe
Great Captains of Antiquity
The Culture of War: Invention and Early Development
The Painful Field: Psychiatric Dimensions of Modern War
No More Heroes: Madness and Psychiatry in War
Military Incompetence: Why the U.S. Military Doesn't Win
To Serve with Honor: A Treatise on Military Ethics and the Way of the Soldier

WITH DONALD BOOSE JR.

Great Battles of Antiquity: A Strategic and Tactical Guide to Great Battles That
    Shaped the Development of War

WITH KAREN S. METZ

A Short History of War: The Evolution of Warfare and Weapons
History of Military Medicine, Vol. 1: From Ancient Times to the Middle Ages
History of Military Medicine, Vol. 2: From the Renaissance Through Modern Times
From Sumer to Rome: The Military Capabilities of Ancient Armies

MAN *and* WOUND
in the ANCIENT
WORLD

*A History of Military Medicine
from Sumer to the Fall of Constantinople*

RICHARD A. GABRIEL

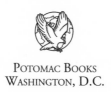

POTOMAC BOOKS
WASHINGTON, D.C.

Library of Congress Cataloging-in-Publication Data
Gabriel, Richard A.
  Man and wound in the ancient world : a history of military medicine from Sumer to the fall of Constantinople / Richard A. Gabriel. — 1st ed.
      p. cm.
  Includes bibliographical references and index.
  ISBN 978-1-59797-848-4 (hardcover)
  ISBN 978-1-59797-849-1 (electronic edition)
  1. Medicine, Military—History. 2. Medicine, Ancient. I. Title.
  RC971.G334 2012
  616.9'8023—dc23

                                                      2011019992

Printed in the United States of America on acid-free paper that meets the American National Standards Institute Z39-48 Standard.

Potomac Books
22841 Quicksilver Drive
Dulles, Virginia 20166

First Edition

10 9 8 7 6 5 4 3 2 1

Contents

1

WAR, WOUNDS, AND DISEASE IN THE ANCIENT WORLD

The information needed to construct a history of military medicine in antiquity is buried in a plethora of nonmedical writings, memoirs of campaigns, personal diaries, and accounts of ancient battles and the military adventures of the heroes of antiquity that have survived and come down to us.[1] Until the eighteenth century when the proper care of the sick and wounded became a regular function of governments, few medical officers or military medical establishments could have been expected to create and preserve information on military medical matters. The task of discovering relevant information about military medicine in the ancient period involves heavily mining the work of classics scholars, historians, and archaeologists who, in their studies of ancient civilizations, brought to light much of the knowledge upon which this book is based. With few exceptions, however, what emerged from these studies was a happy accident. The relevant information concerning military medicine within them was never addressed directly as a subject of historical study.[2]

Military medicine in antiquity, coming from more integrated and far less specialized societies, cannot be properly understood in the context of modern society. Today we distinguish military medicine from medicine that is practiced in the larger society by a civilian medical establishment. The societies of the ancient world made no such distinction. The integrated nature of ancient societies blurred social roles and often retarded the development of scientific and social progress. Thus, the failure of the ancient Egyptians to separate medicine from religion, a separation that the Greek Empirics finally achieved in the third century BCE before falling back into religious influences, strongly

1

retarded the development of empirical medicine during the period when Egypt was at the zenith of its military power. In understanding the ancient world, it is well worth remembering that these societies, in their degree of social differentiation and role specialization, differ from modern society.

The effective practice of military medicine in antiquity depended on a number of factors beyond the era's state of medical knowledge. The presence or absence of these factors was often more crucial to saving a wounded soldier's life than the state of medical knowledge itself. The invention of the tourniquet to stop bleeding and prevent shock, for example, would have been useless had the Romans not also had combat medics and the necessary field transport to move the wounded from the battlefield to field surgical hospitals where doctors could tie off the severed artery. An army's ability to provide combat medics and field ambulances is not related to the state of medical knowledge per se. It relates much more to the degree of organizational sophistication characteristic of the military structure itself. It is impossible to understand military medicine in antiquity without a comprehension of the organizational structure of the army that practiced it.

The primary goal of military medicine, then as now, is to reduce manpower loss caused by enemy action and to save the lives of as many soldiers as possible so they can live to fight again. The medical knowledge available to the military physician is but one element in this larger equation. Military medicine also includes the military doctor's role in conscripting troops for military service. Many of the armies of the ancient world after 2000 BCE were conscript armies. Conscription required that the army pay some attention to the health of the general population, that is, its diet, its mortality rate, and its longevity. An army that accepted anyone would face a medical disaster, so another important role of the military physician was in examining and selecting healthy individuals for military service. The military physician also ensured the safety of food and water supplies, which were also crucial in keeping the army fit for battle. Until modern times, specifically the Russo-Japanese War of 1904–1905, armies suffered far more casualties from diseases caused by contaminated food and water than they did on the battlefield.

Ensuring adequate sanitation in garrison and in the field was among the most important functions of the military physician in the ancient world. Failing to dispose of human waste properly produced outbreaks of disease that rendered armies helpless, a circumstance that has occurred repeatedly even in modern times. Sanitation practices were at their most dramatic in providing that the dead were disposed of properly to prevent contagion, as well as isolating those suffering from disease. As early as 2525 BCE, the Stele of Vultures in Sumer shows military doctors supervising the disposal of the dead in trenches. The book of Leviticus in the Bible spells out the sanitary regulations of the Israelite armies of the first millennium BCE. The priests of the early Israelite armies had the responsibility for training the troops in sanitary practices and enforcing them by military discipline.[3]

The military physicians of ancient armies also had the primary responsibility for maintaining the health of the large corps of animals upon which the army relied for transport. Horses and mules carried diseases that affected humans, so keeping the animals healthy also protected the general health of the army. In 400 BCE, a Greek army fighting on the peninsula of southeastern Greece was rendered incapacitated by an outbreak of dysentery that spread from its animals to the troops. In 1915 CE, an Allied army at Gallipoli was crippled when a similar outbreak of dysentery spread from its mules to the troops.[4] Having little with which to fight disease, the military doctor's best hope of safeguarding the army from disease was to prevent its outbreak in the first place.

The military doctor also played an important administrative role. He was the officer who ensured that the army provided the logistical support to carry out his medical tasks, including arranging adequate transport for moving the sick and wounded in the world's first military ambulances. When the means for transporting the wounded were not available, the army often abandoned wounded soldiers in a nearby village, by the side of the road, or on the battlefield. In some cases, as Alexander the Great did at Sangala, enemy wounded were simply slaughtered.[5] It was not until the appearance of rail transport and the internal combustion–powered vehicle that wounded soldiers could expect medical transport to be available with any degree of regularity.

In a number of ancient armies, most notably the Roman army, the surgeon was the officer responsible for training the army's medical personnel. The notion that the civilian medical establishment could or would provide an adequate supply of trained medical personnel has been obtained only in modern times. Previously, armies trained their own medical personnel, who usually remained separate from any civilian medical establishment. Hippocrates's famous dictum that "war is the best school for the surgeon" suggests only that armies sometimes hired civilian physicians for short periods.

The attempt to construct the history of military medicine in antiquity must encompass a far larger body of information than the medical knowledge that was available to the military doctor at that time. The role of the military physician throughout history also must include his other roles within the larger organizational context of the army in which he served. For most of history, the success of military medicine in preserving the fighting ability of a combat army depended more heavily on the physician's other roles than on his extant medical knowledge per se.

Describing the roles and functions of the military physician will not present the reader with a complete portrait of the development and practice of military medicine in antiquity. It is equally important to understand the nature of warfare in the ancient world as the context within which these descriptions can be correctly understood. Without an accurate picture of the nature of warfare, death, wounding, injury, and disease in the ancient period, a summary of the military surgeon's role would inform to only a limited degree. To understand the role of the military doctor in antiquity, therefore, one must first understand the larger military and medical contexts in which he lived.

The period from 4000 to 2000 BCE was among the most seminal eras in human history. Humans had not yet invented cities or most of the other social structures required to support communal life on a large scale. Agriculture was still in its infancy and could not yet provide an adequate food supply to sustain populations of even moderate size. In any meaningful sense, even warfare itself had not been invented yet. There existed only the embryonic beginnings of a warrior caste, loosely embedded in a tribal social structure that lacked both the physical and psychological requirements to fight wars on any scale. Military technology and organization were primitive, and the professionalization of armies had not yet begun.[6]

The Bronze Age (2500–1200 BCE) changed everything. The Bronze Age saw numerous social, political, economic, psychological, religious, and military innovations emerge that worked to make the conduct of warfare a part of human social existence. In less than two thousand years, humans went from a condition in which warfare was relatively rare and mostly ritualistic to one in which military forces wreaked death and destruction on a modern scale. By the end of the era, warfare assumed truly modern proportions in terms of the size of the armies involved, the administrative mechanisms needed to sustain them, the development and lethality of weapons, the frequency of occurrence, and the scope of destruction achievable by military force that often included the deliberate targeting of civilians and other "nonmilitary" aspects of ancient societies.

What made the birth of warfare possible was the emergence of complex societies with fully developed social structures that provided stability and legitimacy to new social roles and behaviors. The scale of these fourth-millennium urban societies was, in turn, a function of an efficient agricultural ability to produce the resources to feed large populations. These early societies produced the first governing institutions that gave stability and permanence to the centralized direction of social resources on a large scale. At the same time, this centralization demanded the creation of an administrative structure capable of directing social activity and resources toward communal goals. The development of state institutions also gave form and stability to military structures, with the result that the standing army emerged as a permanent part of society. By 2700 BCE, fully developed military structures organized along modern lines were found in Sumer and Egypt.

By the time the Bronze Age gave way to the Iron Age (1200 BCE), humans had further developed their capacity to fight wars. One of the most important stimuli for this military revolution was the discovery and use of iron, which the Hittites most probably first employed as a technology of war.[7] Unlike bronze, which required rare and expensive tin to manufacture, iron was commonly and cheaply available almost everywhere.[8] This plentiful supply made it possible for states to produce enormous quantities of reliable weapons inexpensively. No longer was it only the major powers that could afford standing armies. As the populations of the ancient states increased, the ability to arm larger and larger military forces became possible.

The armies of the Iron Age were the first to practice conscription on a regular basis. No longer limited to defense in times of threat, military service was extended to the need to control large, far-flung empires. The Iron Age gave birth to the national standing army based on citizen service and brought with it a genuine military revolution that changed the nature, scope, and scale of warfare in the ancient world.

During this period, ancient armies invented, perfected, and introduced the prototype of every offensive and defensive weapon used in warfare until the invention of gunpowder in the thirteenth century CE.[9] Evidence of this inventive genius in weapon design appears on the world's first war monument, the Stele of Vultures. Portraying soldiers of the Sumerian king carrying metal-tipped spears and arrayed in a phalanx battle formation, the stele is the first evidence of troop formations in the ancient world. The king himself is shown holding a penetrating ax, the most effective killing instrument of the Bronze Age. The lower palette of the stele depicts a soldier carrying a sickle-sword, its first appearance in history. The king himself is riding in a chariot, which represents the first military application of the wheel. Two important military items of equipment, the metal helmet and body armor, are also shown. Other military monuments of the same period show the socketed bronze ax and the penetrating ax, major developments in killing technology. By 2000 BCE, other Sumerian monuments portray the first appearance of the deadly composite bow. No single army of the ancient world invented and introduced so many new weapons as did the Sumerians.[10]

The ancient solider was well protected by helmets and body armor. Table 1 presents data for the performance characteristics of ancient weapons against the protection offered by armor of the period. With the exception of the socketed penetrating ax, no weapon could be wielded with sufficient muscle-powered force to penetrate the armor of a fully equipped soldier. Ancient armor was so effective that a fully equipped soldier of the ancient world at the battlefield of Waterloo or Gettysburg would have been far better protected from rifle and shell fire than were the soldiers who fought those nineteenth-century battles. The same is true for another military innovation, the helmet. Once the helmet made its appearance, it became a standard item of military equipment until the fourteenth century when modern armies foolishly abandoned it and did not resurrect it until World War I.

Modern studies of skull fractures demonstrate that it takes a minimum of 90 foot-pounds of energy delivered over one square inch to fracture the human skull with a blow delivered to the front of the head.[11] Forty-five foot-pounds of energy will produce a fracture to the temporal-parietal area, and a blow to the zygomatic area requires only 18 foot-pounds to kill.[12] The weapons of the ancient world easily generated these small amounts of energy. But a helmet of

Table 1. *Performance Characteristics of Ancient Weapons*

Weapon	Energy Produced (fpds)[a]	Energy Required (fpds) Bronze[b]	Iron[c]
Gladius (hacking)	101	151	251
Penetrating ax	77	66	110
Sickle-sword	77	245	408
Spear (overhand)	71	137	228
Cutting ax	70	189	314
Eye ax	70	85	141
Javelin	67	99	165
Arrow	47	76	126
Gladius (thrust)	21	182	302
Spear (underhand)	14	137	228

a. **Energy produced** is the energy in foot-pounds delivered by a blow with this weapon by an average soldier.
b. **Energy required (bronze)** is the energy required to cause serious injury when the recipient of the blow is protected by two millimeters of bronze armor or helmet.
c. **Energy required (iron)** is the energy required to cause serious injury when the recipient of the blow is protected by two millimeters of iron armor or helmet.

only two millimeters of metal—at first copper, then bronze, and, ultimately, iron and steel—over a woolen or leather cap effectively neutralized the killing power of any of the ancient weapons except the penetrating ax. The effect of the helmet was to spread the force of the blow over a greater area. With this spreading effect, the force required to fracture the skull is 810 foot-pounds. The most energy that can be produced by a human arm swinging a mace is 101 foot-pounds, and that force is not enough even to render a soldier unconscious.

The data suggest that in the ancient world the balance between killing technology and defensive technology was well struck, with the defense showing a slight advantage. This finding is important because it refutes the commonly held, incorrect notion that the battlefields of the past were scenes of squalid butchery in which every man was at greater risk than those on the modern battlefield. It is important to note that soldiers actually engaged in battle faced good chances of surviving the ravages of ancient weapons. This fact has significant implications for understanding the clinical challenges presented to the military physician.

The armies of the late Bronze Age were quite large. The Egyptian army in the time of Ramses II (1300 BCE) is estimated to have had more than 100,000 men,[13] who were organized into divisions of 5,000 men that could be deployed individually or as a combined force of several divisions.[14] The Battle of Kadesh in 1275 BCE between the Hittites and the Egyptians is the first battle for which relatively reliable strength figures are available. In that battle the Egyptians mounted a four-division force of 20,000 men against the Hittite force of 17,000.[15]

By comparison, however, the armies of the Iron Age were much larger. The Assyrian army of the eighth century BCE comprised at least 150,000 to 200,000 men and was the largest standing military force the world had seen to that time.[16] An Assyrian field army numbered approximately 50,000 men, with various mixes of infantry, chariots, and cavalry.[17] But even the Assyrian army was dwarfed by the Persian armies that appeared three hundred years later. Darius I's army in the Scythian campaign numbered 200,000 men, and the force that Xerxes deployed against the Greeks comprised 300,000 men and 60,000 horsemen.[18] Gen. Percy Sykes's analysis of Xerxes's army suggests that the total force, including support troops, may have numbered a million men, although this number is probably an exaggeration.[19] At the end of the imperial period, the Persians could still deploy large forces. In 331 BCE, when Alexander destroyed the Persian army at the Battle of Arbela, Darius III fielded a force of 300,000 men, 40,000 cavalry, 250 chariots, and 50 elephants.[20]

Philip II of Macedonia could field a combat army of 32,000 men organized in four divisions of 8,192 men each, and the army of Alexander the Great sometimes exceeded 60,000 troops.[21] At the end of the civil wars, Augustus commanded 60 legions, or approximately 700,000 troops. During the imperial period, Roman military forces totaled 350,000 men and routinely deployed consular armies of 20,000 to 40,000 troops. The one exception to the ability of the states of this period to deploy large armies was classical Greece. Being products of relatively small city-states, Greek armies were unusually small even for the Bronze Age. Thucydides recorded that at the beginning of the Peloponnesian War in 431 BCE, Athens could field only 13,000 hoplites, 16,000 older garrison soldiers, 1,200 mounted men, and 1,600 archers. Even these small numbers represented a supreme military effort for Athens in time of crisis.[22]

Sustained by larger populations, cheap and plentiful weapons, the need to govern larger land areas of imperial dimension, and the ability to exercise command and control over larger military establishments, the states of the ancient period produced armies of modern dimensions. Following Rome's collapse in the fourth century CE, few European states were able to muster such sizable military establishments again until well into the nineteenth century.

As the size of armies and the scope of battles increased, ancient armies had to master logistics, or the task of supporting themselves in the field. Changes in the composition of military forces added to their logistics burden. The development of the chariot, for example, required that the Egyptian army maintain repair depots and mobile repair battalions to ensure that the machines remained functional on the march.[23] The Assyrian invention of cavalry squadrons brought into existence a special branch of the logistics train to ensure the army could secure, breed, train, and deploy large numbers of horses. Advances in siege craft required that armies transport siege machinery within their baggage train, and the introduction of artillery, first under the Greeks and brought to perfection under the Romans, added yet another requirement to transport catapults and shot. The need to manufacture and repair the new iron weapons in unprecedented numbers required yet more innovations, such as the mobile blacksmith forge, and the logistics for moving them.

The standard means of logistical transport for Bronze and Iron Age armies was the donkey. In Sumer the solid-wheeled cart drawn by the onager (wild ass) was used early in the period. Ramses II revolutionized Egyptian logistics by introducing the ox-drawn cart, which quickly became the common mode of military logistical transport and was used for almost a thousand years.[24] Xenophon recorded that the normal pack load for a single ox-drawn cart in Greek armies was twenty-five talents, or approximately 1,450 pounds. A mule could carry upward of 200 pounds and a camel approximately 400 pounds. While the oxcart allowed armies to move larger loads, it also slowed the army's rate of movement to a crawl. During this period, there were few packed roads and no paved roads, which the Romans would introduce later. The animal collar had not been invented, and harnesses pressed upon the baggage animals' windpipes, hastening their rate of physical exhaustion. An oxcart could travel two miles an hour for five hours before the animals became exhausted.[25]

The Assyrians' use of the horse gave them increased logistics flexibility, as did the domestication of the camel as a military beast of burden. Using horses in logistics trains increased only slowly under the Persians, finally reaching its height under Philip II of Macedon, Alexander the Great, and, later, the Romans. By the third century BCE, the logistics trains of ancient armies could regularly supply large armies for long periods over great distances. The logistics capabilities of these ancient armies were excellent, and they often managed impressive feats of supply that armies only rarely duplicated before the nineteenth century CE.

The greater strategic mobility of ancient armies that occurred by the end of the Iron Age was a result of the ability of totally integrated societies to produce larger populations and sustain them with the their increasingly sophisticated economies. The strategic range of a typical Bronze Age army was approximately 350 miles by 150 miles. The armies of Sumer and Akkad conducted military operations ranging from the upper Tigris Valley to the city of Ur, or a range of 250 by 125 miles.[26] The Egyptian army of 1400–1250 BCE had a strategic range of 1,250 by 200 miles, or more than twice the range of the armies of the earlier period.

During the Iron Age, Assyria conducted military operations from Assur to Susa and Thebes—an area of 1,250 miles by 300 miles, or five times the range of the Sumerian armies. Persian, Alexandrian, and Roman armies attained strategic ranges typical of modern armies, with the Persian army having a strategic range of 2,500 by 1,000 miles and the Roman armies a range of 2,800 by 1,500 miles.[27] On average, Iron Age armies had a strategic range nine times greater than those of the armies of the Bronze Age. The ability of Iron Age armies to project military power over great distances would not be equaled again until the armies of the nineteenth century were established.

Strategic mobility and range were a function of the ability of ancient societies to place the entire state's resources at the service of their armies. Their ranges also increased as a consequence of improved logistics and staff organization that rationalized planning. The use of naval forces in support of ground operations far from home also augmented their range and flexibility. It is important to remember, however, that ancient armies moved on foot. No army of the modern period equaled or exceeded the ancient armies' rates of movement until the American Civil War, when railroads made faster troop movements possible.

The armies of the late ancient period also made revolutionary advances in tactical mobility and proficiency that had a major impact on the conduct of war. The increased tactical flexibility of small units resulted from a number of factors. For example, the Assyrian army was the first to improve the military footwear of its soldiers. The Assyrian soldier wore a knee-high leather jackboot that had thick leather soles with hobnails to improve traction. The boot also had thin plates of iron sewn into the front to protect the wearer's shins.[28] This boot provided excellent ankle support for troops fighting in cold, rain, and snow and kept foot injuries to a minimum. The new boot was one reason why the Assyrian army could move rapidly over all kinds of terrain in all kinds of weather. Military boots of various designs became standard equipment for the later armies of the period.

Armies also developed all-weather capabilities for ground combat. The Assyrians regularly fought in summer and winter and even conducted sieges in winter.[29] They also fought in marshlands. Placed aboard light reed boats, Assyrian tactical units became waterborne marines and used fire arrows and torches to burn out the enemy hiding among the swamp's brushes and reeds.[30] Mounting military operations in all kinds of weather and terrain became a vital capability for armies of the late ancient period, particularly those of Alexander, Hannibal, and the Roman legions.

The regular use of engineering units also boosted the combat power of tactical units. Persian engineers could divert the course of a river to deprive an enemy fleet of water, a trick they performed in the war against Egypt. Roman military engineering skills reached their height in the ancient period, allowing an army on the march to construct a fortified encampment every night.

The evolution of tactics over nearly fifteen hundred years is a tale of armies boosting their combat power by improving their small-unit tactical capabilities. The results were evident as early as the fourteenth century BCE, when the Egyptian army learned to control large units of different combat capabilities in the first evidence of a combined arms capability. The earliest armies were infantry forces with little in the way of tactical sophistication and could hardly move once arrayed for battle. When infantry formations clashed and one side broke, the victor had no opportunity to pursue the defeated. This situation changed when the Egyptians adopted the chariot.

The chariot introduced the radically new tactical capability of mobility to the battlefield. When equipped with archers armed with the composite bow, the chariot provided the world's first mobile firing platform and was the only weapon that could participate in all phases of the battle with equal effectiveness.[31] The chariot also permitted the first use of mobile reserves committed at a propitious moment to turn a flank or to exploit a breakthrough. Used in different tactical roles, the Hittites' and Assyrians' chariots were bigger and heavier vehicles that were pulled by three horses and carried a crew of three and four, respectively. The Assyrian chariot maximized the role of shock rather than mobility by attacking enemy infantry formations from several directions at once. Once engaged, the crews dismounted and fought as infantry. The Assyrians were the first to use mounted infantry, and their use of the chariot strongly resembled that of armored personnel carriers in modern times.

A major Assyrian innovation was the invention of cavalry. The spur and stirrup had not yet made their appearance, and Assyrian cavalrymen used the saddle girth, crupper, and breast strap to stabilize the rider. Pressure from the rider's leg and heel of his boots controlled the horse. This development made possible the first use of mounted archers, or the famed "hurricanes on horseback" mentioned in the Old Testament. The ability of the horse to traverse uneven terrain made cavalry forces especially lethal in the pursuit and valuable for reconnaissance and providing flank security, two new tactical capabilities. By the time of Cyrus the Great, the Persian army's ratio of cavalry to infantry was 20 percent cavalry to 80 percent infantry, for the largest cavalry force in the world.[32]

The Greeks discovered the secret of heavy infantry. The heavily armored hoplite soldier fighting in tightly packed phalanxes had the advantage of being almost impervious to cavalry attack. Its major disadvantage, however, was its inability to maneuver and to conduct pursuit. Philip II of Macedonia made the phalanx heavier. He also armed the densely packed formations of the Macedonian phalanx with a fifteen-foot-long pike called the *sarissa*, which weighed twelve pounds.[33] Philip's tactical contribution was to reduce the role of infantry as the primary striking and killing arm of the Greek army. He used his heavy infantry formations as a platform for maneuver of his primary striking arm, the heavy cavalry armed with the long *xyston* lance and deadly *machaira* sword.[34] Philip was the first to use cavalry as the primary combat arm of an ancient army.

The tactical proficiency of ancient armies went through several phases. Beginning with the primacy of infantry, the Egyptians' use of the chariot introduced the new element of mobility to the battlefield. The Assyrians found a new role for the chariot as mounted infantry, but they relied more on their cavalry to provide mobility and flexibility. The Persians' reliance on cavalry led to their neglect of heavy infantry, and Philip's use of heavy infantry formations as a platform of maneuver signaled the leading role of cavalry as the primary striking force of ancient armies. In each phase of tactical development, the role of infantry as the main maneuver and killing element on the battlefield declined. How much more surprising, then, that the next major army to appear on the ancient battlefield found its strength in the maneuverability and killing power of heavy infantry while relegating cavalry to a secondary role.

The spine of the Roman legion was its heavy infantry formations, whose tactical proficiency and lethality were not surpassed for almost fifteen hundred years. The secret of the Roman killing machine was a soldier who was the first to fight within a combat formation while remaining tactically independent of its movement as a unit. He was also the first soldier in history to employ primarily the *gladius* (sword) instead of the spear.[35] The Roman gladius caused more deaths on the battlefield than any other weapon until the invention of the firearm.[36]

The infantry formations of earlier armies were packed masses of men pressed against one another with no spacing between individual soldiers or units. The Roman innovation built in spaces between soldiers and units, greatly increasing their flexibility and mobility. The spacing between each soldier was sufficient to allow independent movement and fighting room within an area of five square yards, or enough space for the soldier to wield his sword. Soldiers were assigned to sixty- to eighty-man units called maniples, each one laterally separated from the next by twenty yards, or a distance equal to the frontage of the maniple itself. The maniples were arrayed in staggered lines, with the second and third lines covering the gaps to their front. Each line of infantry was separated from the next by an interval of approximately a hundred yards. This resulting quincunx, or checkerboard formation, allowed tactical flexibility for each maniple and enabled it to deliver or meet an attack from any direction.

The resurgence of infantry as the primary tactical killing arm inevitably reduced the cavalry to a secondary role. Roman infantry ruled supreme in the ancient world until its defeat at the Battle of Adrianople in 378 CE. Its defeat at the hands of barbarian cavalry shook the tactical thinking of the ancient world. Followed by a hundred years of invasions by tribal cavalry armies, the empire's collapse in the West was attributed to the superiority of cavalry over infantry. The death of disciplined infantry and the primacy of cavalry were also consequences of the social and military superiority of the new European tribal states. If there had been any doubt in the mind of tactical thinkers about the role of cavalry, the Battle of Hastings in 1066 CE, in which a cavalry army massacred an infantry force, settled the question for hundreds of years. During the Middle Ages, the armored knight became the prototype of the successful warrior, and infantry all but disappeared from the battlefield.

Both siege craft and artillery came into existence to confront the fortified city, the most powerful defensive system produced in the ancient world. The first undisputed example of a fortified city was Uruk in Mesopotamia, dating from 2900 BCE.[37] The city's walls enclosed an area of 5.5 square miles. To place this development in perspective, Athens, after the expansion under Themistocles, covered an area of 2.5 square miles, while Jerusalem in 43 CE enclosed an area of only 1 square mile. Even the city of Rome at the time of the emperor Hadrian in the first century CE was only twice as large as the city of Uruk, built more than three thousand years earlier.[38]

Fortified cities put armies at great risk. Safe behind the city's walls, defending armies could live off well-stocked provisions for long periods while attacking armies were forced to live off the land until hunger, thirst, and disease ravaged their ranks. No army bent on conquest could force a strategic decision as long as the defender refused to give battle. A conquering army that bypassed fortified strong points placed itself at risk of attack from the rear. No successful army could prevail without the ability to overcome fortifications. One of the earliest inventions used to defeat fortifications was the battering ram, dating from at least 2500 BCE.[39]

The Assyrian armies of the eighth century BCE were masters of siege craft. The key was to coordinate several types of assault at different points on the walls simultaneously. Battering rams supported by siege towers were brought into position at several locations along the walls. At the same time, scaling ladders with lever crews were deployed at other places. Sappers and tunnelers worked to weaken and collapse a section of the walls' foundation. At the appropriate time, scaling ladders were used to mount attacks over the walls in several places at once to force the defenders to disperse their forces.[40] The idea was quickly to mass more soldiers at the point of entry than the defender could bring to bear. As a general rule, a city could mount about 25 percent of its population to defend against an attack. Thus, a city of thirty thousand people could muster about eight thousand men to defend against an attacking force that easily exceeded thirty thousand to forty thousand soldiers. The advantage almost always rested with the besieging army.[41]

The steady development of siege craft reached new heights during the reigns of Philip II of Macedon and Alexander the Great. Philip realized that the new Macedonian army would obtain only limited objectives if it was not provided with the capability for rapidly reducing cities. Philip introduced the use of sophisticated siege operations to his army, copying many of the techniques the Assyrians first used and that the Persians passed to him.[42] The Romans' ability to reduce fortifications was probably the best in the ancient world, but they relied more on organization and application than on engineering innovation. For the most part Roman siege engines were improved versions of Greek and Persian machines.[43]

Philip II of Macedon established a group of artillery engineers within his army to design and build catapults. Of this period the most important contribution of Greek engineering to warfare was the invention of artillery in the form of catapults and torsion-fired missiles. The earliest example, dating from the fourth century BCE, was called a *gastraphetes* (literally, belly shooter) and was a form of primitive crossbow that fired a wooden bolt on a flat trajectory along a slot in the aiming rod.[44] Later, weapons fired by torsion bars powered by horsehair and ox tendon (the Greeks called this material *neuron*) springs could fire arrows, stones, and pots of burning pitch along a low parabolic arc. Some of these machines were quite large and mounted on wheels to improve tactical mobility. One of them, the *palintonon,* could fire an eight-pound stone more than three hundred yards, a range greater than that of the Napoleonic cannon.[45] While Philip first used them as weapons of siege warfare, Alexander later employed them as covering artillery. Alexander's army carried prefabricated catapults that weighed only eighty-five pounds. It dismantled larger machines and brought them along in wagons.[46]

Roman advances in the design, mobility, and firepower of artillery produced the largest, longest-range, and most rapid-firing artillery pieces of the ancient world. It was not until the American Civil War that an artillery piece could fire a longer distance than a Roman one, and still it fired shot that weighed less than Roman shot. No artillery piece could fire faster than the Roman guns until the invention of the first breech-loading artillery gun in 1875. Roman catapults were much larger than Greek models and were powered by torsion devices and springs made of sinew kept supple in canisters of oil. If we are to believe Flavius Josephus in his account of the Roman siege of Jerusalem in the first century CE, the largest of these artillery pieces, the onager (called the wild ass because of its kick), could hurl a hundred-pound stone four hundred yards.[47]

The Roman writer Flavius Vegetius noted that each legion had ten *onagi*, one per cohort, organic to its organization.[48] Smaller versions of these machines, such as the scorpion, were compact enough to be transported by horse and mule, and could fire a seven- to ten-pound stone ball more than three hundred yards.[49] Smaller machines fired iron-tipped bolts. Designed similar to the later crossbow but mounted on small platforms or legs, these guns required a two-man crew. As the world's first rapid-fire field guns against enemy formations, they fired twenty-six-inch bolts over a range of almost three hundred yards, with a rate of fire of three to four rounds a minute.[50]

The weapons of the ancient world were effective in the hands of a competent soldier. In determining the risk of death and wounds faced by the ancient soldier, it must be kept in mind that the soldier's chances varied greatly depending on the army in which he fought and at what point in history he saw combat. The Egyptian soldier fighting the Hyksos, for example, had little chance of escaping death or injury, while the Roman soldier fighting against the Belgae had a very good chance of escaping injury altogether.[51] Modern battles see a fair share of dead and wounded on both sides, but in ancient battles the vanquished suffered horribly while the victor less so. At the Battle of Marathon in 490 BCE, for example, the Athenians suffered less than two hundred dead out of a force of ten thousand hoplites. At Issus, Alexander's army endured only two hundred dead while inflicting fifty thousand casualties upon the Persians; and at Cynoscephalae, the Romans killed eight thousand Greeks, virtually destroying the Macedonian army at a cost of only seven hundred men.[52]

It is often thought that battles involving masses of men in close combat were horrifically bloody. In fact, as long as the units remained engaged and intact, they were rarely so. When arrayed in a close-order infantry phalanx, only the first two ranks could actively engage in any fighting and then not for very long. Estimates are that the lines of the phalanx could remain engaged for not more than ten minutes before exhaustion took its toll.[53] Moreover, most of the combat power of the packed phalanx could not be brought to bear upon the killing. When the front lines came together, only the second rank could move into the spaces in the first line and engage the enemy. If the infantry was armed with the spear and shield, as was the case in all armies until the Roman army of the third century BCE, the ability to wield one's weapons against the enemy press was considerably reduced.[54] As long as the phalanx held together, the tactics, weapons, and formations limited the infantry's ability to kill on a great scale.

The real killer on the ancient battlefield was fear.[55] As stress increased, the probability that someone would lose his nerve and run increased. Sometimes the actions of a single soldier caused panic in a unit or an entire army. A phalanx would suddenly shatter and take flight, as the once cohesive fighting force became a mob of terrified human beings trying to escape. Soldiers fled in all directions, often casting away their weapons, shields, and armor. Because armies had little means to engage in lethal pursuit, fleeing the battlefield often worked to limit casualties. The introduction of the chariot and then the spear and archer cavalry changed the battlefield dynamic. Fleeing soldiers became easy targets, and the pursuit, once a rare event, developed into the primary means of totally annihilating a defeated army. Killing as they went, chariots and cavalry rode through and around the fleeing mob and herded it back toward the center, where the victors sometimes spent all day killing the defenseless. Unless the victorious commander ordered a halt to the killing, it often happened that an entire army would be mercilessly slain.

Table 2 presents manpower and casualty data for fourteen battles fought between 2250 and 45 BCE by the armies of Sumer, Persia, classical and imperial Greece, tribes, and the Romans. The dates of the battles range over two thousand years, allowing us to account for changes in more lethal killing technology as it affected casualty rates. It must be said, however, that there is no way to verify the accuracy of these numbers extracted from classical literature. It is probable, however, that at least the proportions between the figures are nearly accurate.[56] The data indicate that the percentage of dead (killed in

Table 2. *Combat Death Rates of Ancient Armies*

DATE (BCE)	BATTLE	ADVERSARIES		NUMBER OF TROOPS		NUMBER KILLED		% DEFEATED KILLED IN ACTION
		VICTOR	DEFEATED	VICTOR	DEFEATED	VICTOR	DEFEATED	
2250	***	King of Akked	Ur	5,400	13,500	***	8,040	59.5
334	Granicus	Alexander	Memnon	36,000	40,000	125	10,000	25.0
333	Issus	Alexander	Darius III	36,000	150,000	200	50,000	33.0
331	Arbela	Alexander	Darius III	40,000	340,000	300	100,000	29.4
237	Metaurus River	Hamilcar Barcas	Mercenaries	10,000	25,000	***	6,000	24.0
218	Trebia	Hannibal	Sempronius	50,000	40,000	few	20,000–30,000	50.0
216	Cannae	Hannibal	Varro	50,000	80,000	5,500	70,000	87.5
202	Zama	Scipio Africanus	Hannibal	50,000	50,000	2,000	20,000	40.0
197	Cynoscephalae	Flamininus	Philip V	20,000	23,000	700	8,000	34.7
168	Pydna	Aemillus Paullus	Perseus	30,000	44,000	***	20,000	45.4
102	Aquae Sextiae	Marius	The Teutons	40,000	100,000	300	90,000	90.0
86	Chaeronea	Sulla	Archelaus	30,000	110,000	14	100,000	90.9
48	Pharsalus	Caesar	Pompey	22,000	45,000	300	15,000	33.0
45	Munda	Caesar	Pompey	48,000	80,000	1,000	33,000	41.2

action) suffered by a defeated army was on average 37.7 percent of the total force. Death rates for victorious armies, however, were considerably lower, or about 5.5 percent of the force. Even with a technological advantage in weapons, it was still necessary to kill at close range, and the gross disparity in kill rates suggests strongly that most of the killing occurred after one side broke and could be hunted down and slain with comparative ease.

If the battles are analyzed in terms of those that matched a tactically and technologically superior army against an inferior army, it seems that these factors made an important difference in casualty rates. The six battles that met these conditions were Alexander's battles against the Persians at the Granicus River, Issus, and Arbela; the Roman battles against the Macedonian Greeks at Cynoscephalae and Pydna; and the Roman battle against the tribal armies of the Teutons at Aquae Sextiae. In these battles, the tactically and technologically superior force killed 42.6 percent of the enemy force, inflicting 5 percent more casualties than could normally have been expected. The advantage is also reflected in lower casualty rates for the victorious armies. Alexander's armies suffered only 0.5 percent average death rates in the three battles against the Persians, while the Romans endured a 1.3 percent death rate against the Greeks and Teutons. Armies relatively equal in tactics and weapons could expect to see 5.5 percent of their forces killed in action. On average, then, superior armies suffered a death rate of only 2.4 percent, its superior tactics and equipment conveying a force multiplier of more than 100 percent.

Except for some surviving Roman and Assyrian records, we have only limited data on the number of wounded in ancient battles. If, however, we know the size of the defeated army and subtract the number of soldiers killed in action and taken prisoner, we are left with a rough approximation of the number of wounded. Since slightly wounded men would have probably been taken prisoner, we may suppose that the number of wounded reflects those injured severely enough to be worthless to the slave buyers. Table 3 presents the data for the number of wounded and prisoners for the six battles for which information is available. Approximately 35.5 percent of the defeated army could expect to suffer wounds serious enough to allow them to be left on the battlefield. When added to the 37.8 percent of the vanquished who were killed, no less than 73.3 percent of the men who took the field could expect to be killed or wounded before the day was out.

Table 3. *Calculation of Wounded in Ancient Battles*

BATTLE	TOTAL FORCE	KILLED	TAKEN PRISONER	WOUNDED	
				Number	*Percent*
Granicus	40,000	10,000	20,000	10,000	25.0
Metaurus River	25,000	6,000	2,000	17,000	68.0
Zama	50,000	20,000	20,000	10,000	20.0
Cynoscephalae	23,000	8,000	5,000	10,000	43.4
Pydna	44,000	20,000	5,000	19,000	43.2
Pharsalus	45,000	15,000	24,000	6,000	13.3

There is no certain way to measure the victor's number of wounded. The ratio of dead to dead in each army, if the proportion held, would indicate a wound rate to the victorious army of 5.8 percent. If kill and wound rates were generally low while the forces were locked in combat, owing to the factors noted earlier, then a wound rate of 5.8 percent for the victor does not seem high. Donald Engels's analysis of Alexander's armies suggests that the victorious Macedonians suffered approximately five wounded for every dead.[57] The Roman army's medical system planned for a wounded casualty rate of between 2 and 10 percent, or an average of 6 percent. The data suggest that seven of every ten soldiers of a defeated force would become casualties by day's end, while the victors could expect to lose one in every ten men either killed or wounded. Only the wounded in the victorious army were fortunate enough to receive medical attention.

By comparison, data from examinations of the kill and wound rates for the U.S. Army as a percentage of engaged strength, while controlling for staff and logistics support as noncombatants, appear in table 4. A modern conventional army could expect to suffer 17.6 percent of its force killed in action and another 41.8 percent wounded. Almost six of every ten men on the modern battlefield could expect to become casualties. It is worth pointing out, however, that the figures in table 4 are for wars in which the U.S. Army was victorious. If we compare these rates with those of victorious armies of the ancient period, the disparity is striking. A victorious ancient army could expect to suffer only 5.5 percent dead compared to 17.6 percent for a modern force. An ancient army would suffer only 6 percent wounded compared to 41.8 percent

Table 4. *Casualties as a Percentage of Engaged Strength*

WAR	ENGAGED STRENGTH	KILLED IN ACTION		WOUNDED	
		Number	*Percent*	*Number*	*Percent*
Civil War	700,000	67,058	9.6	324,893	46.4
World War I	500,000	116,516	23.3	204,002	40.8
World War II	1,714,285	405,399	23.6	670,846	37.1
Korea	240,000	33,629	14.0	103,040	42.9

for a modern army. Thus, a soldier in a victorious army in modern times has a three times greater chance of being killed and a seven times greater chance of being wounded than his ancient counterpart did. In defeat, the chances of a modern soldier being wounded are only 6 percent greater than that of a similar soldier in ancient armies.

It is interesting to note the type and nature of wounds most commonly suffered by soldiers in ancient armies. The *Iliad* provides the oldest literary account of battle wounds suffered by these soldiers, and Franz H. Frölich's analysis provides baseline data on battle wounds of the ancient Greek period.[58] Table 5 shows a profile of the wounds described in the *Iliad* by type of weapon, number of impact, and degree of mortality. Of the 147 wounds recorded by Homer, 114, or 77.7 percent, resulted in fatalities. The areas of greatest lethality were the head and chest, which still account for most battle wound fatalities today. Of the thirty-one wounds to the head, all were fatal.[59] This fatality rate compares to that of the Crimean War, in which 73.9 percent of head wounds resulted in death. The percentage of fatal head wounds in the Civil War was 71.7 percent.[60] During World War I, head wounds without dural penetration had a lethality rate of 10 percent, while wounds that produced dural penetration had fatality rates of 35 percent.[61]

Of all the weapons examined in the *Iliad,* arrows accounted for less than 10 percent of the wounds that the soldiers suffered and resulted in the lowest mortality rate, or 42 percent. This outcome occurred because of a combination of factors. An arrow fired from a composite bow could not penetrate the body armor of the day, and the unarmored parts of the body offered a small target area. The most likely place for an arrow wound to occur was in the

Table 5. *Wounds and Fatalities in the* Iliad

Type of Weapon	Number	Mortality (%)
Spear	106	80
Sword	17	100
Arrow	12	42
Sling	12	66
	N=147	114 or 77.6%

extremities, in the upper arms and legs, and in the neck. Arrow wounds to the neck were usually fatal. Because of their greater target area, wounds to the arms and legs were much more common. Frölich notes that 16 percent of the wounds described in the *Iliad* were to the upper and lower extremities.[62] These wounds would have caused fatal shock or massive bleeding only if an artery were severed. Except for the neck, arteries are located deep in the body, are protected by bone and tissue, and are difficult to hit. One suspects, therefore, that arterial wounds were rare. The data on arterial wounds extrapolated from modern wars suggest that these wounds were relatively uncommon. Although the penetrating power of rifle bullets and artillery fragments is much greater than that of arrows, only 0.29 percent of the wounded in the Civil War suffered arterial wounds.[63] In World War I, the rate was 0.40 percent, in World War II 1.0 percent, and in the Korean War 2.4 percent.[64] There is no reason to believe that the probabilities of inflicting this type of wound on the ancient soldier were greater.

Blood loss and shock killed most men on the ancient battlefield. It was Roman military physicians who invented ligature, or the art of tying off an artery to stop bleeding. In World War II when ligature was widely practiced, 59 percent of the soldiers who underwent ligature and survived required the amputation of a limb.[65] Amputation was not practiced by ancient doctors until Roman military physicians introduced it; however, it is unlikely that ligature and amputation would have helped very much. In the Civil War the overall mortality rate produced by surgical amputations averaged 40 percent. In the early days of the war, the mortality rate was as high as 83 percent.[66]

The most common wound suffered by the ancient soldier was the broken bone. Ancient Egyptian and Sumerian medical texts discuss broken bones extensively. The first evidence for the use of a splint applied to a broken bone is seen in mummies in ancient Egypt. However, since Egyptian physicians were proficient at skull surgery, it is not unreasonable to expect that they were also familiar with the simple technique of setting a broken bone. One reason why fractures may have been common among the casualties of ancient armies is that they are so easy to inflict. With the exception of the skull, there is very little difference in the amount of force needed to fracture the various bones in the human body. Even the thickest bones of the upper leg require only marginally more force to fracture than do the thinner bones of the forearm. On average, 67.7 foot-pounds of impact energy will produce a fracture of any bone in the human body except the skull.[67] Every one of the close combat weapons of the ancient world could easily generate this amount of force.

The pattern of fractures in ancient battles can be determined by reconstructing the body movements of the soldier in close combat. These experiments show that the clavicle, or collarbone, was probably the most commonly broken bone. Almost any overhand blow with any weapon could strike the clavicle with sufficient force to break it. A body blow with a stabbing spear to the armor plate protecting the sternum would easily fracture the breastbone, and a side blow to the chest would cause a broken rib. The arms were among the most vulnerable areas. Most armor did not cover the upper and lower arms, leaving them defenseless against slashing cuts and fractures. The forearms were usually protected by leather or bronze greaves, but the force of a downward slash with an ax or gladius could readily fracture the forearm or wrist. Up to the nineteenth century CE, the cavalryman's most common injury was the broken wrist.[68]

If an arrow struck an artery or vein without causing death by shock or bleeding, the chances of contracting a lethal infection were great indeed. In World War II when sulfa and penicillin were available, 49 percent of the cases of arterial wounds resulted in gas gangrene.[69] In 62.1 percent of the cases, arterial wounds resulted in amputation.[70] The chances of dying from an infected wound in antiquity were no greater than that faced by any soldier in any war until at least the early days of World War I when immunization and, later, the large-scale production of penicillin in 1942 increased the soldier's chances of survival. The wounded soldier in the ancient world was at risk of wound infection from the same three microbiological threats that threaten the modern soldier: tetanus, gas gangrene, and septicemia.

The tetanus bacterium is endemic to soil and is found in the richly manured soil typical of the agricultural societies and battlefields of the ancient world. It is common where sanitation is poor, and human and animal waste is present. If a soldier's wound was not thoroughly cleansed with water, soap, or wine, or was sutured or bandaged too quickly or tightly, resultant tetanus infection was almost a certainty. The ancient medical practice of leaving a wound open for several days before closing it with sutures or bandages produced far fewer tetanus infections than the practice of rapid closure that was employed after ancient times until the early days of World War I.

Since there was no way to prevent tetanus infections until the introduction of immunization in World War I, it is likely that the rates of tetanus infections in ancient armies were equivalent to those found in armies up to the early twentieth century. If the rates of tetanus infection for the Peninsula War, Crimean War, Civil War, Franco-Prussian War, and early World War I are examined, the average rate of tetanus infection for battle wounds was 5.6 percent, with a mortality rate of 80 percent.[71] In neither ancient nor modern times was there any effective mechanism for treating the infection once it began.

Gas gangrene presented another deadly threat. Until the middle years of World War I, the average rate of gas gangrene among wounded soldiers was 5 percent. With treatment, the survival rate among British forces was 28 percent. In ancient times gangrenous wounds produced almost total mortality.[72] The ancient medical practice of repeatedly cleansing a wound for several days before closure would have done much to reduce the onset of gangrene infection. Until the Boer War, British military doctors routinely bandaged or sutured wounds as soon as they could get to the wounded soldier. This system resulted in high death rates from gangrene as necrotic tissue remained in the wound. By the middle years of World War I, British physicians began leaving the wound open for several days and then cleansing it several times before closing it with stitches or bandages. The rediscovery of this ancient medical technique resulted in a decline in the gangrene mortality rate from 28 percent to 1 percent.[73]

Septicemia, or blood poisoning, presented a third threat to the wounded soldier. Blood poisoning occurs when the common body bacteria staphylococcus enters the blood stream. Wounds to arteries and major veins offer a major risk of septicemia. The rate of such wounds is approximately 1.7 percent.[74] In modern times the introduction of antibiotics made it possible to combat blood infection. But before World War II, any soldier with a septicemic infection usually died.

If the data on wound mortality and infection are combined, a rough statistical profile of the causes of wound mortality for the ancient soldier can be produced. Of a hundred soldiers wounded in action, 13.8 percent would die of shock and bleeding within two to six hours of being wounded. Another 6 percent would contract tetanus, and 80 percent of them would die within three to six days. Five percent would see their wounds turn gangrenous, and 80–100 percent would die within a week. Approximately 1.7 percent would contract a septicemic infection, and 83–100 percent would succumb within six to ten days. On average, then, 25 percent of wounded soldiers would die of their wounds within a week to ten days. By comparison, the average death rates from all wounds in the Crimean War was 20 percent, while the rate for the Civil War was 13.3 percent. Throughout history, these same four factors— shock and bleeding, tetanus, gangrene, and septicemia—remained the major causes of death among the wounded until the closing years of World War I.

The health of an ancient society's general population placed limits upon the quality of soldier its army could obtain, and these limits formed the medical parameters within which diseases occurred that affected military operations. The general health of the populations of the ancient world was better from the Middle Bronze Age (2500 BCE) to the end of the Greek classical period (323 BCE) than it would ever be again until the beginning of the twentieth century.[75] The decline in average life span began in the late Neolithic period (6000 BCE) after agriculture introduced changes in man's diet and groups' population densities. The growth of urbanization greatly increased contagion patterns. The decline in health leveled off between the Middle Bronze Age and the classical period.

In the Neolithic period, the average life span was 35.4 years. By the end of the Early Bronze Age, it had declined to 32.1 years. By the Middle Bronze Age, it had increased to 34.7 years and reached its peak in the classical period at 38.1 years.[76] Note that the figures are averages and are depressed by a child morality rate averaging from 49.8 to 55 percent at various times in the ancient period.[77] Of every one hundred children born, half died before age five.[78] Of the fifty survivors, twenty-seven died before age twenty-five; of the twenty-three survivors, nine died by age thirty-five; of the remaining fourteen, six lived to age fifty; and only three lived to see sixty.[79]

The decline began again in the Hellenistic period and continued through Roman times. In the fourth to third centuries BCE, the average age of death for adults was 42.4 years. A century later during the Roman period, the average age of adult death was 38 years.[80] This demographic drop was a lasting one. Not until the second half of the nineteenth century did demographic indexes reach the levels of the classical age.[81]

There is little doubt that the general health of the populations of the ancient world left much to be desired by modern standards. For most of the time, however, the general health of European populations was no better. During the Middle Ages and the Industrial Revolution, overcrowding, polluted water supplies, unhygienic burial practices (owing largely to the Christian religions of the period, which invented the concept of hallowed burial ground and insisted on burying the dead within the walls of the city), poor nutrition, and industrial pollution produced populations considerably less healthy than those of the cities of the ancient world.

For most people in the West, their general health has improved more since the mid-twentieth century than in the preceding three millennia. But not always. An American medical team examining the inhabitants of three Greek villages between 1957 and 1962 found the villagers suffering from the following medical conditions: malaria, typhoid fever, amoebic dysentery, pulmonary tuberculosis, scrofula, diabetes, jaundice, hepatitis, pneumonia, meningitis, diphtheria, undulant fever, scarlet fever, cataracts, and other eye diseases. Additional ailments included a range of acute respiratory diseases, gastrointestinal disorders, rheumatic pains, nutritional dystrophy, high blood pressure, tonsillitis, peptic ulcers, hernia, gout, and sciatica. This medical profile strongly resembles the medical reality that would have confronted a Greek physician of the early fifth century BCE.[82]

Still, it was possible for ancient armies to fill their ranks with initially healthy individuals. There were, however, many health risks presented by military life itself. In ancient armies, as with all armies until the Russo-Japanese War of 1904–1905, more soldiers died from disease than from enemy weapons. The Union Army in the Civil War assembled the first accurate records of losses to disease. The Union Army lost 110,065 men to enemy fire and 224,586 to disease during four years of war.[83] The Russo-Japanese War was the first war in which more soldiers were lost to hostile fire than to disease. In that war, the Russian army lost 709,587 men to battle wounds and only 7,960 to disease. The figures were repeated on the Japanese side, where 21,802 men were lost to enemy fire and only 5,877 to disease.[84] This reversal in loss rates from disease is regarded as a major watershed in the history of military medicine.

Disease outbreaks in ancient armies were most likely to occur when large numbers of men were assembled for long periods out of garrison where normal, if primitive, sanitary facilities were not available. Aside from the Egyptian and Roman armies that routinely took great care in the field to construct sanitation facilities and segregate them from water and food supplies, most armies took no precautions at all. Greek field armies, for example, provided no common sanitary facilities and used whatever areas were handy when the need arose. Xenophon tells us that sentries in Spartan camps moved only a little way from their posts to relieve themselves. The failure to provide adequate sanitary facilities continued for both military and civilian populations until modern times. During the Middle Ages, the floors of castle garrisons were covered with straw to absorb the urine and feces routinely deposited by the inhabitants in any convenient spot. In urban areas up to the nineteenth century, the chamber pot was the most common method of domestic sanitation, and, well into the 1870s, people routinely emptied its contents each morning into the public streets. Indeed, the primary impetus for the creation of forested urban parklands in cities was to provide places where people could relieve themselves with some degree of privacy. Armies on the march probably had less chance of epidemic, however, since they moved away from infection sites. The most likely place for a devastating outbreak of disease was in siege operations, where large numbers of people lived in proximity amid poor sanitary and nutritional conditions. It was also common practice to catapult human and animal corpses over the walls to cause a disease outbreak among the defenders.

Most descriptions of diseases in ancient literature are not precise enough to allow their identification with certainty. Historians, for example, cannot determine if the Great Plague described by Thucydides that killed a quarter of the Athenian population was caused by typhoid.[85] The decimation of Rome's population in the second century CE suggests an outbreak of smallpox, but diagnosticians cannot be certain. Some diseases, such as cholera and bubonic plague, have relatively recent origins and can be safely omitted from those af-flictions that beset ancient armies. Others, such as dysentery, typhus, malaria, snail fever, typhoid, and small pox, can be asserted with confidence to have struck armies of the ancient world.[86]

The most common disease of ancient armies and indeed throughout his-tory was dysentery, which was commonly called campaign fever. The first de-scription of dysentery appears in Egypt in the Ebers Papyrus around 1550 BCE.[87] Dysentery is accurately described in the writings of Hippocrates, and Roman medical texts outline hygienic practices for preventing its outbreak. The disease afflicted the armies of the Middle Ages almost routinely and caused more deaths during the Crusades than Saracen arrows did. It has been called "the most dangerous and pervasive disease in human history."[88]

Ingesting food and water that is contaminated with a waterborne bacillus causes dysentery. Human and animal excrement are excellent sources of trans-mission. During sieges, the lack of waste disposal facilities, improper washing of hands, and infected water supplies caused frequent outbreaks. While some variants of the disease have a 50 percent mortality rate, the usual rate does not exceed 5 percent.[89] The infection immobilizes large numbers of soldiers who cannot fight for periods of two to three weeks. Some idea of the impact of a dysentery outbreak on a combat force can be gauged from the fact that while 81,360 Union Army personnel died from the disease, twenty times that num-ber, or 1,627,000 troops, contracted it during the war.[90]

Typhoid fever is caused by the bacterium *Salmonella typhi*, which lives in the human digestive tract and is transported by human feces. The disease is contracted by ingesting contaminated food and water supplies, and the same factors that give rise to dysentery also cause outbreaks of typhoid fever. The common housefly, drawn to exposed feces, can rapidly transmit the disease to the human food supply. The Assyrians thought that evil spirits caused illness and used the symbol for the common housefly for those spirits that caused disease.[91] Roman engineering manuals specified that all latrines be dug to a depth of three meters and be covered with wood or stone caps to keep sun-light away from the depository so that flies would not be drawn to the feces and spread disease.[92] No other army of the ancient world seems to have taken similar precautions.

An army caught in the midst of a typhoid outbreak was rendered useless as a combat force. The mortality rate of 10–13 percent was high, and the disease, with its pain and delirium fever, required four weeks to run its course.[93] In the Napoleonic wars, 270 of every 1,000 men who caught the disease died.[94] In the Crimean War, it was a more common cause of death than was enemy fire. During the Boer War, the British lost 13,000 men to typhoid, and another 64,000 victims of the disease were invalided home. By contrast, only 8,000 men were lost to enemy fire.[95] During the Spanish-American War, 90 percent of American units shipped to Cuba suffered outbreaks of varying severity, and 20 percent of the entire U.S. forces caught the disease.[96] In ancient times, the disease was probably epidemic and not endemic.

Typhus is among the most common and deadly diseases associated with armies throughout history. It is caused by an organism midway between a bacterium and a virus that lives on the blood of animals, including rats. It is transmitted by a number of insect vectors, but the most common is the human body louse, *Pediculus humanus*. Living in humans' clothes and hair, it transmits the disease as it moves from one human to another. A disease of crowded humanity, typhus is found in jails, on ships, in armies, and in overpopulated housing conditions.

The disease produces fever, chills, and aching joints accompanied by severe headache. After the fourth or fifth day, skin lesions begin forming on the extremities. Patients become disoriented and deranged. The mortality rate is generally 10–40 percent, but it has been known to kill entire armies.[97] In Napoleon's winter campaign in Russia, the disease decimated his army. In the city of Vilnius, Lithuania, Napoleon abandoned 30,000 typhus cases; almost all died.[98] During World War I, no fewer than 2,500 cases were being admitted a day on the eastern front in 1915. During the Russian Civil War (1917–1921), it is estimated that 25 million Russians were struck by the disease, of whom 2.3 million to 3 million died.[99] Typhus is a disease of temperate zones, and the armies of Greece and Rome were probably familiar with it.

Smallpox outbreaks were probably fairly common in the ancient world. The earliest provable case of the disease occurred in 1145 BCE when Ramses V of Egypt died of it.[100] Smallpox was among the most feared of ancient diseases because of its tendency to blind, cripple, and scar the victim. It is likely that many ancient accounts of outbreaks of leprosy were really epidemics of smallpox. The great Antonine Plague, which struck Rome in the second century CE, was probably caused by smallpox-infected legions returning from the eastern provinces.[101] The disease comes in a number of varieties, some of which produce mortality rates upward of 90 percent. The more common strains produce death rates of 20–40 percent.

Until the late nineteenth century when advances in the theory of contagion, immunization, and antibiotics finally began to reduce death rates, disease remained as much of a scourge of modern armies as it was for ancient armies. It is impossible to arrive at any precise death rates for armies of the ancient world resulting from disease. In terms of expected rates, however, an ancient army struck by an outbreak of dysentery could expect to lose 5 percent of its force to the disease. If struck by typhus, 10–40 percent of the force would die, typhoid would claim 10–30 percent, and smallpox 15–40 percent. While the epidemic raged, the army was defenseless and utterly incapable of mounting combat operations.

An army in the field suffers considerable manpower loss to injury. In World War I, the Allied armies on the western front lost almost six thousand men a month to accidents, falls, accidental wounds, frostbite, trench foot, and heatstroke. An army on the march can expect to lose a considerable percentage of its combat force in the act of moving to the battlefield. Moving an armed force of ten thousand men is no easy task, and the march takes a heavy toll on the soldiers' health. Ancient armies moved in column for the same reason that nineteenth-century armies did: the column was the best way to maintain organizational integrity and control. An army moving in column ten abreast often took hours to pass a single point. Not counting baggage animals and animals carrying provisions, Alexander's army of sixty-five thousand men and six thousand cavalry, when arranged in column ten abreast, stretched for 16.5 miles.[102] The column formation itself caused injuries. The air breathed by the men in the center of the formations was putrid. The dust choked their nostrils, irritated their eyes, and congested their lungs. In a single day, nosebleeds, eye irritation, and respiratory problems would cause such severe injuries that men would drop out of the ranks and be left behind. In severe heat and cold, the injury rate increased dramatically.

Malnutrition was a major problem. Modern armies estimate that a 160-pound soldier carrying a moderate load for eight hours requires 3,402 calories and seventy grams of protein a day.[103] However, the stress and effort of combat field operations increase the amount of food required to keep the soldier healthy and functioning. In desert or semiarid climates, especially those with high temperatures and low humidity, the soldier requires a minimum of nine quarts of water a day. These minimal nutritional requirements will keep the soldier functioning for only a few days. If nutritional requirements are kept at this level over a march of seven to ten days, many soldiers would be unable to fight, even if they suffered no additional injuries or health impairments.

The diet of the ancient soldier was barely sufficient for sustained military activities. Their field diet consisted mostly of grain—wheat, barley, or millet—ground into flour to make bread, biscuits, and porridge. The standard ration was between 2.2 and 3 pounds of grain per soldier per day. But when wheat is milled and baked, its caloric and protein content are reduced. Thus, 2.2 pounds of wheat turned into bread produces only 2,500 calories and a hundred grams of protein. The digestive process, however, does not make full use of even these reduced amounts. When 2.2 pounds of wheat are milled, cooked, eaten, and digested, the body realizes less than 2,025 calories and eighty grams of protein. If the same amount of wheat is made into porridge, it produces only 1,000 calories.[104] An ancient army on the march for more than three to four days consistently lost its strength as the soldiers' health and stamina declined with each day. It is not difficult to imagine a considerable portion of the army melting away on the march because of nutritional reasons. In cases where water and food were in short supply, the entire army might wither and die from hunger and thirst.

In hot climates, the soldier was vulnerable to heatstroke. Carrying sixty pounds amid conditions of high temperatures and low humidity aggravated by constant dust and breathing putrid air could easily cause a soldier to succumb to heat exhaustion. Sunburn was also a problem. Roman soldiers protected themselves from sunburn by applying palm or olive oil. A Roman account provides an excellent example of what could happen to a field army that did not take precautions to protect itself from the heat. In 24 BCE Aelius Gallus, the Roman governor of Egypt, lost almost his entire army and at least one complete legion to thirst and heatstroke while conducting operations in Arabia. Many of the survivors suffered permanent damage and had to be mustered out of service.[105]

Some idea of the loss rates that ancient armies experienced in the field can be surmised from the results of a U.S. Marine Corps experiment conducted in the Twentynine Palms desert training area in 1984.[106] Although the troops in the exercise were provided with the best nutrition, clothing, and shelter; more than sufficient water; frequent rest periods; and precise instructions on how to conserve body energy, over a fifteen-day period 110 men out of 6,476 in the study had to be hospitalized for heat exhaustion. Another 53 became combat ineffective from debilitating headaches induced by the heat, 31 were hospitalized for severe body cramps and nausea, 46 suffered nosebleeds from the dust, and another 46 were hospitalized for eye irritations though they had been given protective eye goggles.[107] In all, 286 men were lost to heat-related illnesses even though the exercise required no sustained marching.

Ancient armies suffered many of the same injuries that plague modern armies and that make a soldier a casualty, including accidents, falls, contusions, cuts, bruises, sprains, and broken bones. In the Marine study, more than 1,101 men suffered some injury serious enough to require medical attention at the battalion aid station or evacuation to other medical facilities. Two hundred and twenty-eight Marines suffered blisters, lacerations, and abrasions; and 169 were injured by some "general trauma" serious enough to take them out of the field. Another 152 had irritations of the nose and throat, and the category of "other injuries" accounted for 337 men requiring medical treatment.[108] No less than 17 percent of the total force required medical treatment or hospitalization for injuries sustained on an exercise that lasted only fifteen days.

Ancient armies also fought in cold climates. The Assyrian incursions into Armenia and Kurdistan required fighting in snow, rain, and freezing temperatures. Roman armies fought in Germany, Italy, the Alps, eastern Europe, and the mountains of Spain, all of which have climates that challenged the survivability of soldiers even in World War II. Xenophon recorded in the *Anabasis* that he almost lost his entire army in the mountains of Turkey when the men slept unprotected and awoke to a snowstorm.[109] Sometimes cold weather caused tremendous casualties. Alexander crossed the Hindu Kush with 100,000 men and arrived on the other side thirteen days later with only 64,000, for a loss rate of 36 percent. Hannibal managed to cross the Alps but at terrific cost: his army of 38,000 infantry and 8,000 cavalry lost 18,000 infantrymen and 2,000 cavalry to the weather by the time it reached Italy.[110] During Napoleon's retreat from Moscow, all but 350 of the 12,000 men of the Twelfth Division died of the cold. In World War II, only 15 percent of soldiers injured by the cold could be returned to service, suggesting that most cold injuries then and now were serious indeed.[111]

An army on the march was a potential medical disaster. At the minimum, an army of 10,000 men could expect to lose 4 percent of its force to heat-stroke or exhaustion. Cold produced much higher injury rates. Another 1,700 men, or 17 percent of the force, would be lost to routine injuries. As the army moved along, its general resistance to disease declined. The dust from the marching column choked the soldiers' lungs, dried out their sinuses, and produced chronic coughing, blinding headaches, and severe nosebleeds. Blisters from the leather thongs and boots were endemic. In extremes of hot or cold, many soldiers died. Others would be so damaged that their health would be impaired for the rest of their lives.

Notes

1. Franz Hermann Frölich's major work *Die Militärmedicin Homer's* (Stuttgart: Enke, 1879) contains all the citations found in classical literature dealing with military medicine. The articles are organized by chapter and verse, and include all the major works of antiquity from Homer and the Bible through Livy, Caesar, and other Roman writers up through the Dark Ages.

2. The only complete history of military medicine from ancient times to the present remains Richard A. Gabriel and Karen S. Metz, *A History of Military Medicine,* 2 vols. (Westport, CT: Greenwood, 1992).

3. Richard A. Gabriel, *The Military History of Ancient Israel* (Westport, CT: Praeger, 2003), 92–93.

4. Fielding H. Garrison, *Notes on the History of Military Medicine* (Washington, DC: Association of Military Surgeons, 1922), 38. For some idea of the risk to humans from horses in ancient armies, see U.S. Army, Mounted Service School, Fort Riley, KS, *The Army Horse in Accident and Disease* (Washington, DC: U.S. Government Printing Office, 1905).

5. Lucius Flavius Arrianus (Arrian), *The Campaigns of Alexander,* trans. Aubrey de Selincourt (London: Penguin, 1958), book 5, paragraph 24, line 7.

6. Richard A. Gabriel, *The Culture of War: Invention and Early Development* (Westport, CT: Greenwood, 1990), 35–37.

7. Clarence H. Long, "Metallurgy," *Encyclopaedia Britannica,* 15th ed. (Chicago: Encyclopaedia Britannica, 1985), 350.

8. Ibid.

9. Yigael Yadin, *The Art of Warfare in Biblical Lands in Light of Archaeological Study,* trans. M. Pearlman, 2 vols. (New York: McGraw-Hill, 1963), 36–40.

10. Richard A. Gabriel and Karen S. Metz, *From Sumer to Rome: The Military Capabilities of Ancient Armies* (Westport, CT: Greenwood, 1991), 25–30.

11. Charles W. Gadd and John P. Danforth, *A Study of Head and Facial Bone Impact Tolerances* (Warren, MI: General Motors Corporation, 1969), 7.

12. Ibid. See also Harold M. Frost, *Orthopaedic Biomechanics* (Springfield, IL: Charles C. Thomas, 1973), 198, for the force figures required to break human bones other than the skull.

13. Robert J. Wenke, *Patterns in Prehistory: Mankind's First Three Million Years* (New York: Oxford University Press, 1980), 486. For a detailed analysis of the Egyptian army in antiquity, see Richard A. Gabriel, *Empires at War: A Chronological Encyclopedia*, vol. 1 (Westport, CT: Greenwood, 2005), chapter 3.

14. Arthur Ferrill, *The Origins of War: From the Stone Age to Alexander the Great* (London: Thames and Hudson, 1985), 58.

15. A detailed examination of the structure, weapons, and capabilities of the Egyptian army can be found in Richard A. Gabriel, *Thutmose III: The Military Biography of Egypt's Greatest Warrior King* (Washington, DC: Potomac Books, 2009), 49–65.

16. Ferrill, *The Origins of War*, 58.

17. T. N. Dupuy, *The Evolution of Weapons and Warfare* (Indianapolis: Bobbs-Merrill, 1980), 10.

18. These numbers are taken from Plato's account of the war and are considerably less than those found in Herodotus.

19. Sir Percy Sykes, *A History of Persia* (London: Macmillan, 1955), 1:196–98.

20. Robert Laffont, *The Ancient Art of Warfare* (New York: Time-Life, 1966), vol. 1, 45. These figures cannot be taken as entirely accurate. Arrian tells us that Darius had 40,000 cavalry, 100,000 infantry, 240 chariots, and "a few elephants." Curtius puts the number of cavalry at 45,000 and the infantry at 200,000. Justin says Darius's total force was 500,000, and Diodorus says he had 800,000 infantry and 200,000 cavalry.

21. Dupuy, *Evolution of Weapons and Warfare*, 14.

22. Laffont, *Ancient Art of Warfare*, 73.

23. Yadin, *Art of Warfare in Biblical Lands*, 1:89.

24. R. O. Faulkner, "Egyptian Military Organization," *Journal of Egyptian Archaeology* 39 (1953): 41–47.

25. Army Veterinary Department, *Animal Management* (London: War Office, 1908), 299.

26. Laffont, *Ancient Art of Warfare*, 1:46, chart 3.

27. The calculation of the strategic range of the Roman army is my own, using the same formula as found in ibid.; however, Laffont does not provide figures for the Romans.

28. Ibid., 45.
29. H. W. F. Saggs, "Assyrian Warfare in the Sargonid Period," *Iraq* 25, part 2 (Autumn 1963): 145–46. Saddam Hussein attempted to exterminate these same "marsh Arabs" by draining the swamps and marshes of the lower Tigris and Euphrates Rivers in order to expose them to ground attack.
30. Yadin, *Art of Warfare in Biblical Lands*, 2:303.
31. Gabriel, *Culture of War*, 95.
32. Yaha Zoka, *The Imperial Iranian Army from Cyrus to Pahlavi* (Tehran: Ministry of Culture and Arts Press, 1971), 19.
33. Richard A. Gabriel, *Philip II of Macedonia, Greater than Alexander* (Washington, DC: Potomac Books, 2010), 93–94. See also Peter Connolly, *Greece and Rome at War* (Englewood Cliffs, NJ: Prentice-Hall, 1981), 78–79.
34. Gabriel, *Philip II of Macedonia*, 107–8.
35. Robert L. O'Connell, "The Roman Killing Machine," *Quarterly Journal of Military History*, Autumn 1988, 37–38.
36. Ibid.
37. James Mellaart, *The Neolithic of the Near East* (New York: Scribner, 1975), 50–58. See also Majid Khadduri, "Sumerian Civilization," *Encyclopaedia Britannica*, 15th ed. (Chicago: Encyclopaedia Britannica, 1985), 21:950.
38. Hans J. Nissen, *The Early History of the Ancient Near East, 9000–2000 B.C.* (Chicago: University of Chicago Press, 1988), 72.
39. Yadin, *Art of Warfare in Biblical Lands*, 1:55, 147.
40. Ibid., 2:313–28, for a description of Assyrian siege tactics.
41. Ibid.
42. For an account of Greek siege machinery, see J. K. Anderson, "Wars and Military Science: Greece," in *Civilization of the Ancient Mediterranean: Greece and Rome,* eds. Michael Grant and Rachel Kitzinger (New York: Scribner's, 1988), 1:330–38. See also Gabriel, *Philip II of Macedonia*, 125–29.
43. Ernest Dupuy and Trevor N. Dupuy, *The Encyclopedia of Military History from 3500 B.C. to Present* (New York: Harper & Row, 1986), 28–30. See also Graham Webster, *The Roman Imperial Army of the First and Second Centuries A.D.*, 3rd ed. (Totowa, NJ: Barnes & Noble, 1985), 240–43.
44. Dupuy and Dupuy, *Encyclopedia of Military History*, 29.
45. Ibid.
46. Ibid.
47. Ibid. See also Flavius Josephus, *The Jewish War*, trans. G. A. Williamson (London: Penguin, 1984), book 5, 6.3.
48. Flavius Renatus Vegetius, *On Roman Military Matters: A 5th Century Training Manual in Organization, Weapons, and Tactics, as Practiced by the Roman Legions*, trans. John Clarke (London: Red and Black Publishers, 2008), book 2, 25.

49. Dupuy and Dupuy, *Encyclopedia of Military History*, 25.

50. Ibid. See also Richard A. Gabriel, "Trajan's Column," *Military History*, September 2010, 26.

51. The Hyksos were armed with the sickle-sword, composite bow, penetrating ax, and the chariot, weapons unknown to the Egyptians at the time. They were also equipped with helmets and body armor. For much of the imperial period, the Romans fought tribal armies that were inferior to them in almost every way, a situation that resulted often in great slaughter.

52. Laffont, *Ancient Art of Warfare*, 101.

53. Ibid., 103. On the endurance of men in battle, see Philip Sabin, "The Mechanics of Battle in the Second Punic War," in *The Second Punic War: A Reappraisal*, eds. Tim Cornell, Boris Rankov, and Philip Sabin (London: Institute of Classical Studies, University of London, 1996), 70–78.

54. Christopher Matthew, *A Storm of Spears: A Reappraisal of Hoplite Combat* (London: Pen and Sword, 2010), 96–98.

55. For a history of psychiatric collapse in war, see Richard A. Gabriel, *No More Heroes: Madness and Psychiatry in War* (New York: Hill and Wang, 1988). See also Charles Jean Jacques Joseph Ardant du Picq, *Battle Studies: Ancient and Modern Battle*, trans. John Greely and Robert C. Cotton (Harrisburg, PA: Military Service Publishing Company, 1947).

56. Some of the figures in this table are taken from Laffont, *Ancient Art of Warfare*, 101. Others are taken from accounts of the battles in ancient literature.

57. Donald W. Engels, *Alexander the Great and the Logistics of the Macedonian Army* (Berkeley: University of California Press, 1978), 151.

58. Frölich, *Militärmedicin Homer's*, 56–60.

59. Ibid.

60. E. Stephen Gurdjian, "The Treatment of Penetrating Head Wounds of the Brain Sustained in Warfare: A Historical Review," *Journal of Neurosurgery* 39 (February 1974): 165. The statistics for Civil War casualties used herein are from James McPherson, *Ordeal by Fire: The Civil War and Reconstruction* (New York: Knopf, 1982), 149–80; and *Historical Statistics of the United States* (Washington, DC: Department of the Census, 1975), 1140.

61. Gurdjian, "Treatment of Penetrating Head Wounds," 165.

62. Frölich, *Militärmedicin Homer's*, 59.

63. Peter A. Aldea and William Shaw, "The Evolution of the Surgical Management of Severe Lower Extremity Trauma," *Clinics in Plastic Surgery* 13, no. 4 (October 1986): 565–66.

64. Ibid.

65. Ibid.

66. Ibid.

67. Frost, *Orthopaedic Biomechanics*, 198.

68. Christopher Duffy, *The Military Experience in the Age of Reason* (New York: Atheneum, 1988), 227–28.

69. Aldea and Shaw, "Evolution of the Surgical Management," 565–66.

70. Ibid.

71. Basic information on the diseases addressed here can be found in *The Professional Guide to Disease* (Springhouse, PA: Intermed Communications, 1982).

72. Aldea and Shaw, "Evolution of the Surgical Management," 561.

73. Ibid.

74. Ibid., 558.

75. Mirko D. Grmek, *Diseases in the Ancient Greek* World, trans. Mireille Muellner and Leonard Muellner (Baltimore: Johns Hopkins University Press, 1989), 104.

76. Ibid., 99.

77. Ibid., 100.

78. Gabriel and Metz, *From Sumer to Rome*, 28.

79. William S. Barnett, "Only the Bad Died Young in the Ancient Middle East," *Journal of International Aging and Human Development* 21, no. 2 (1985): 155–60.

80. Grmek, *Diseases in the Ancient Greek World*, 104.

81. Ibid.

82. Roderick E. McGrew, *Encyclopedia of Medical History*, with Margaret P. McGrew (New York: McGraw-Hill, 1985), 103.

83. Ibid.

84. Ibid.

85. Thucydides, *History of the Peloponnesian War*, trans. M. I. Finely (London: Penguin, 1972), book 2, 47.4. For typhoid as the cause of the plague, see Stephan Berry, "Genes of the Phalangites: Bioarchaeology and the Ancient Battlefield," *Ancient Warfare* 4, no. 2 (2010): 46–47.

86. The best work on ancient diseases remains Don Brothwell and A. T. Sandison, *Diseases in Antiquity: A Survey of the Diseases, Injuries, and Surgery of Early Populations* (Springfield, IL: Charles C. Thomas, 1967).

87. Ibid., 104.

88. Ibid.

89. Ibid., 352.

90. Ibid., 313.

91. Garrison, *Notes on the History of Military Medicine*, 28. The Mesopotamian god of death and disease was Nergal.

92. Webster, *The Roman Imperial Army of the First and Second Centuries A.D.*, 259–60.

93. McGrew, *Encyclopedia of Medical History*, 348–49.

94. Ibid.

95. Ibid.

96. Ibid.

97. Ibid., 313.

98. Ibid.

99. Ibid.

100. R. J. Doyle and Nancy C. Lee, "Microbes, Warfare, Religion, and Human Institutions," *Canadian Journal of Microbiology* 32, no. 3 (March 1986): 195. The mummy of Thutmose III (1504–1450 BCE) shows signs of what might have been smallpox scars. See Gabriel, *Thutmose III*, 4–5.

101. Ibid.

102. Engels, *Alexander the Great and the Logistics*, 54.

103. Richard A. Gabriel, *Soldiers' Lives through History: Antiquity* (Westport, CT: Greenwood, 2007), chapter 5 "Rations," 31–38.

104. Ibid.

105. Saul Jarcho, "A Roman Experience with Heatstroke in 24 B.C.," *Bulletin of the New York Academy of Medicine* 43, no. 8 (August 1967): 767–68.

106. Morris Kerstein and Roger Hubbards, "Heat Related Problems in the Desert: The Environment Can Be the Enemy," *Military Medicine* 149 (December 1984): 650–56.

107. Ibid., 653.

108. Ibid., 654.

109. Alan Steinman, "Adverse Effects of Heat and Cold on Military Operations: History and Current Solutions," *Military Medicine* 152 (August 1987): 389.

110. Richard A. Gabriel, *Hannibal: The Military Biography of Rome's Greatest Enemy* (Washington, DC: Potomac Books, 2010), 150–51.

111. P. Byron Vaughn, "Local Cold Injury—Menace to Military Operations: A Review," *Military Medicine* 145, no. 5 (May 1980): 306.

2

THE ORIGINS OF
MILITARY MEDICINE

Medicine emerged at a point in human development when humans came to believe they could do something to prevent or cure the illnesses, injuries, and diseases that afflicted them. The initial incursions into a primitive doctrine of prevention were closely bound with religion and myth, and involved spells, incantations, sacrifices, and other forms of submission to unseen higher forces. Early humans believed that deities, angered by sin, broken taboo, immoral habits, or failure to observe religious rituals, caused illness and disease. Conforming to the gods' will was perceived as the only way to achieve good health.[1] One reason why ancient societies respected old age was that they viewed longevity as a result of the gods rewarding a good moral life by permitting the virtuous to live longer.[2] The first stirrings of humanity's desire to control its own destiny arose with the belief that humans had the means to control their own health, if only by conforming to the gods' wishes. It was no accident that the practice of medicine was associated with the religious priesthood in ancient times. As primitive as it may seem, the belief in one's ability to placate the deities constituted the first doctrine of disease prevention, without which further progress in medicine would not have been possible.

More evidence exists from ancient civilizations about the conduct of war than about the physicians and medicine that accompanied the combatants. Writing and record keeping emerged shortly after 4000 BCE in Sumer and slightly later in Egypt, but most of the extant written medical records appeared relatively late in the ancient period. What survived from the earlier periods is fragmentary. Cuneiform, hieroglyphics, and Linear A and B were administrative writing systems and differed from the spoken languages of the day. It was not until the classical period in Greece around 700 BCE that the first written language generally used by the populace made its appearance. As such, the accounts of medical practice are far more complete for late Greece and Rome than for Sumer, Egypt, and Assyria. Evidence of military medical practice in the earliest periods must be pieced together from a few surviving medical records, the historical literature, archaeological artifacts, and an understanding of the nature of the general social, economic, and military order that attended ancient societies.

The nature of medical care available to the soldiers of the earliest armies of Sumer, Egypt, and Assyria depended heavily on the general state of medical knowledge extant in the society of which the army was a part. This connection seems logical enough, but it was not always the case, especially in later societies. During the Roman imperial period, for example, the state of medical knowledge was shaped largely by military practice, which slowly seeped into the general Roman society. Until then, Roman civilian medicine had manifested an abysmally low level of medical knowledge and technique. Although the practice of medicine remained in the grip of a powerful priesthood, Egyptian military physicians' experience with war wounds played an important part in Egyptian medicine. Paradoxically, at the time when Egypt was reaching the pinnacle of its military power, Egyptian medicine was plunging into its mystical phase. This new emphasis, however, did not prevent Egyptian military physicians from practicing clinical battlefield medicine.

The successful application of a society's general level of medical knowledge to the soldier was largely a function of the organizational sophistication of the army in which he fought. Well-organized armies, for example, those of Rome and Assyria, developed formal military medical establishments that were able to deliver relatively good medical care to their soldiers. Other less organizationally developed armies, such as those of classical Greece, made it impossible for them to develop an adequate military medical service. Part-time Greek citizen armies, which required only marginal training and skills, did not fight far from home and thus did not require medical services any more than they required logistics trains or siege craft. The latter two additional capabilities also failed to develop as a result of the general primitive organization of the classical Greek armies. The same may be said of later Arab armies.

Given that medical care was no less important to the ability of an army to fight, survive, and continue military operations in ancient times than it is today, it is curious that ancient writers did not pay more attention to it in their written commentaries. This oversight is especially puzzling given that kings and their apologist scribes went to great lengths to record their military exploits. Perhaps the lack of direct evidence of military medicine is because it was so commonplace and not considered important enough to write about, in much the same way that hardly anyone today produces great literary or historical works on military administration or the quartermaster corps. Or, conversely, perhaps ancient military medicine was so poor and ineffective that writing about it would have belittled the otherwise glorious accomplishments of the rulers.

Most medical histories in the West begin with the assertions that Hippocrates was the father of modern medicine and the Greeks were the first to practice truly empirical medicine. While it is true that the Greeks were the first to write in a commonly understood and readable language and produced a number of medical texts that have had the good fortune to survive, it is incorrect to regard the Greeks as the source of modern clinical medicine or as the innovators of military medicine. The survival of the Greek and Roman medical texts depended on Muslim physicians, not Western doctors, who reintroduced these texts to Europe as a consequence of the Arab invasions of the Middle Ages. Then the texts themselves had to be retranslated from Syriac back into Greek and Latin.[3]

The history of empirical medicine is at least twenty-five hundred years older than classical Greece and in the case of sophisticated surgery almost eight thousand years older. By the classical period, the state of Western medical knowledge in general and military medicine in particular had declined considerably from that found in the more ancient civilizations. Despite Herodotus's claim that Egyptian medicine had advanced to a high state in his day, at the time Herodotus wrote, Egyptian medicine had declined to the lowest point in its history, entering a mystical phase and turning its back on a two-thousand-year tradition of clinical medical pragmatism. By the time of Alexander the Great some two centuries later, Egyptian medicine had changed again, this time abandoning its mystical influence and turning once more toward empiricism. But this development was more the result of Egyptian contact with the new Empirics of Greece rather than the other way around.[4] To the degree that Egyptian medicine appeared to the Greeks of Herodotus's time to be high art is testimony to the generally low level of Greek medicine of the day. The level of military medical care available to the Sumerian (2500 BCE), Egyptian (1700 BCE), and the Assyrian (900 BCE) soldier was superior to that which attended the hoplite warrior of classical Greece.

The modern age tends to dismiss the effectiveness of the medical treatments that ancient physicians, priests, and sorcerers used as being little more than spells, rituals, and incantations. This lack of regard is the result of the modern emphasis on a mechanical model of medical practice that is itself less than two hundred years old. Yet today's physicians have often come to realize the importance of a patient's psychic state in the healing process. Almost all armies of the world retain chaplains who administer religious rituals to the wounded and dying. Wounded men identify battle nurses with the security of their mothers, and even the most severely wounded men receive comfort from the nurses' words of hope. Modern medicine itself has given birth to a subdiscipline that seeks to integrate empirically based therapies with positive psychic states. Some research suggests that psychic activity can create disease-specific antibodies within the immune system. The modern medical establishment's attempts to rejoin the physical with the psychic phases of medical treatment are regarded today as a major medical advance. It may be wise to recall that all ancient physicians practiced this unity as a matter of course.

Ancient medicine is sometimes disparaged because of the perception that most ancient beliefs constituted a poor theory of medicine. Indeed, because ancient medicine lacked an accurate theory of contagion or even an accurate portrait of human anatomy, it is assumed that this knowledge gap could only lead to poor medical practice. It was, after all, the first rule of Hippocrates that a physician should do no harm. This view of ancient medicine, however, overlooks the fact that the ancient soldier often had a much better chance of surviving a battlefield injury than did his later counterparts, at least until World War I. The use of incantations or spells for minor wounds, for example, did not require the healer to touch and probe them as the medical mechanics of all armies routinely did through at least the Civil War. Without the accompanying practice of sterilization, the probe probably did more to infect wounds than any other medical implement, whereas the ancient spells and incantations reduced the probing of the wound and consequent spread of infection.

Moreover, the practice of washing a wound several times before closing it, a technique first used in Sumer, or bandaging it only loosely until it began to heal, a common practice in Egypt, did much to reduce the initial rates of tetanus and gangrene that resulted from battle wounds. From the Middle Ages to World War I, as noted in chapter 1, the most common medical procedure for treating wounds was to bandage them immediately and tightly. The practice proved disastrous in the Boer War and produced tetanus rates of 28 percent. During the later days of the war when the practice was abandoned and the ancient technique was used instead, tetanus rates dropped to 1 percent.[5]

To regard ancient medical practice as inadequate because its general theories of medicine were incorrect overlooks the fact that modern medicine has often been premised on theoretical views that were later proven to be erroneous. The use of radical surgery for breast cancer, for example, was based on a thoroughly incorrect theory of tumor transmission, though it often succeeded for other reasons. The chemical and hormonal theories that underlay thousands of useless hysterectomies were equally incorrect. There is, as yet, no adequate theoretical basis for electroconvulsive therapy even though it is often the only successful treatment for deep depression. The list of disproved theories could be greatly expanded. In the same way that erroneous medical theory has done little to stop the practice of clinical medicine in the modern age, however, there is no reason to believe it did so in the ancient world either. This observation is especially true for those military physicians who had to deal with critical and immediate medical problems on the battlefield.

Nor did the lack of medical theory prevent the development in ancient times of highly empirical, pragmatic, and effective medical protocols for treating specific conditions and injuries. The first surgery for which we have evidence is trephining of the skull. The procedure involved drilling or scraping a hole through the skull to expose the dura, the layer of tissue covering the brain. While we may be sure that ancient physicians believed they had good reason to embark upon such a dangerous and sophisticated operation, we know little of those reasons today. One assumption is that trephining was done to allow evil demons (or other types of pressure) to escape. Trephining was practiced in many cultures as long ago as the eighth millennium BCE. A team of trained pathologists conducted a comprehensive study of trephined skulls drawn from these various cultures and from different periods and revealed the amazing conclusion that the survival rate for this operation among ancient peoples was almost 100 percent.[6] Even allowing for methodological difficulties associated with the size of the sample and questions about using evidence of replacement bone growth to measure survival rates, the success rate appears remarkable. By contrast, until 1870 the survival rate for skull surgery that was performed by Western physicians, guided by modern medical theory, and accompanied by some antisepsis and anesthesia was almost zero.[7] Whatever other variables may have been at work in the practice of trephining, lacking an accurate theory of general medicine clearly did not prevent ancient physicians from developing an effective medical procedure for opening the skull that permitted the patient to survive.

Another example of a useful ancient procedure can be drawn from Egyptian medicine of the second millennium BCE. The direct evidence for Egyptian skull surgery is found in documents dating to 2000 BCE, but an analysis of the hieroglyphs used in these documents suggests that the documents incorporate medical knowledge at least a thousand years older.[8] Despite the Egyptians' poor knowledge of human anatomy, such as the belief that all major vessels of the body were filled with air and terminated at the anus, they nonetheless developed a successful surgical procedure for treating linear and depressed skull fractures. The technique is modern in every respect and involves incising the scalp, peeling it back, separating the depressed fragment from its surrounding tissue with a flattened probe, elevating the fragment to relieve pressure on the dura, and bandaging the skull in a manner that allowed the incision to heal normally.[9] In a civilization that did not use the helmet for almost twenty-three hundred years after it first placed an army in the field and where the skull-shattering mace was the primary weapon, Egyptian military physicians—despite their poor medical theories—had plenty of opportunities to clinically address the problem of skull fractures.

Medical practice in the ancient world was given an enormous stimulus from the frequent wars that attended all the major ancient civilizations. In Sumer, for example, the rival city-states were constantly at war with one another for almost a thousand years. Sargon II, the great Assyrian warrior-king

(725–701 BCE), carried out no fewer than ten major wars of conquest or suppression in less than sixteen years. Between 890 and 640 BCE, the Assyrian state conducted 108 major and minor wars, punitive expeditions, and other significant military operations against neighboring states.[10] Whatever else war provided, it gave military physicians frequent opportunities to experiment with new treatment techniques until they found something that worked.[11] As is still the case with military medicine today, the emphasis of ancient military medicine was more on achieving clinical results than on gaining theoretical insight.[12] Armies are pragmatic social institutions that are quick to adopt whatever works and abandon what does not. That armies of the ancient world and their military physicians should have been any less practical seems unlikely.

The military doctor attending an ancient army had an advantage that his modern-day counterpart often does not: the former did not encounter a gross difference between wounds encountered in civilian life and those found on the battlefield. Indeed, the disparity is a relatively modern distinction for the medical practitioner and came about only after the invention of high-speed projectiles and chemical explosives. Only in the last 150 years has a civilian doctor gone to war and expected to treat wounds with which he was not familiar in his civilian practice. Indeed, the distinction continues to operate today, only in reverse. Because of the availability of modern automatic weapons to the civilian population, civilian doctors in large urban trauma centers often confront injuries that were heretofore seen only on the battlefield. In what must rank among medical history's paradoxes, the U.S. Army now sends its military physicians to urban trauma centers for clinical training in dealing with battle wounds.[13]

For ancient physicians, the wounds encountered on the battlefield would not have been remarkably different from those they routinely encountered in civilian practice. The cuts, bruises, fractures, and even gaping flesh and muscle wounds produced by ancient weapons would have appeared commonplace to the ancient physician. Fractures of the legs, arms, wrists, and skull, for example, were all familiar to civilian doctors of ancient Egypt. People living in a culture next to a river suffered these types of fractures routinely, as people wearing sandals commonly slipped on wet ground. Pathological evidence indicates that the most common fractures among ancient Egyptians were those of the wrist and arm, precisely the same kinds of injury Egyptian infantry forces often suffered while attempting to ward off blows from enemy weapons.[14] It is no accident that the first evidence for the use of the splint is found in ancient Egypt.[15]

Skull, chest, pelvis, and lower leg fractures with attendant paralysis that soldiers commonly suffered while engaged in siege operations were familiar to physicians who attended large gangs of corvée laborers constructing the tombs, dikes, pyramids, ziggurats, and other massive public works characteristic of the civilizations of the ancient world. Even gaping flesh and muscle wounds caused by a hacking sword had a serious counterpart in Egyptian civilian medical practice: crocodile bites. An Egyptian medical book, the *Book of Bites,* records examples of people mutilated by crocodile bites in the Nile and provides a protocol of treatment for the resulting gaping wounds. Lions and other big cats were common in Sumer and Assyria, and the armies of these countries trained their soldiers by having them fight the animals. The resulting teeth and claw wounds provided yet another opportunity for training physicians. Unlike civilian doctors drafted for military service on short notice in modern times, the military physicians of ancient armies would have encountered few wounds on the battlefield that were unique to their civilian clinical experience.

This account is not to suggest that ancient medical practice was more effective than modern practice, for it usually was not. Yet until modern times the risk to the wounded soldier was equal to or even greater than that faced by the ancient soldier. And remarkably in so many instances ancient physicians were correct in their attribution of the causes of clinical diseases. The Sumerians and Assyrians, for example, were experts at recognizing the onset of liver disease. The clay models of livers from ninth-century BCE Assyria were more anatomically correct than those used in Europe, even after the Middle Ages.[16] The Assyrians also introduced urinalysis as a diagnostic tool. This technique was so impressively effective that when the Muslims introduced the Syriac medical texts describing it into Europe, the urine flask became the symbol of the medical profession in Europe.[17] The rabbis of Israelite armies of the thirteenth century BCE served as a sanitary corps and were experts at the detection and prevention of disease and contagion. The Hebraic tradition of kashruth ensured an uncontaminated food and water supply, and the ritual butchering of animals by *shochets* (religiously trained slaughterers) made them experts at recognizing the clinical signs of human and animal sickness. The shochet originally was employed to ensure that an animal sacrifice was fit to offer the gods. Later, he extended his skills to examining the food supply for the army, a practice that reduced illness and disease considerably.

The contention here is that the general level of treatment and medical practice available to the ancient soldier was often adequate for dealing with the battle wounds and injuries he was most likely to suffer. Like military physicians throughout history, the military physicians in ancient armies emphasized pragmatic and effective treatments based on hard clinical observation and experience rather than on proven medical theory. In a number of respects, the level of medical care available in some ancient armies, most notably the Roman army, was not surpassed in the modern era until World War I. For most of history after the fall of Rome, however, the soldier received more primitive and less effective field medical care than he had received in earlier times. Not surprising, the death rates for the wounded were also higher.

While most armies of the ancient world had some physicians attending the wounded, the presence of military doctors was more readily apparent in some armies than in others. It must be noted that the information about the nature of the military medical establishment in any ancient army is premised upon a knowledge of the surviving archaeological evidence. In the Egyptian army, for example, we may be relatively confident that military physicians were stationed in the major garrisons of the empire. The Assyrians seem to have developed the prototype of a modern military medical service or at least to have produced the world's first military medical professionals. The Greeks, for all their emphasis on an empirical approach to medicine, did little to establish a medical service for their citizen armies, while the Romans employed a medical corps that was truly modern by any standard. The presence of doctors on the battlefields in some of the more ancient armies—those of Sumer and Akkad, for example—must remain to some degree a matter of conjecture. But the Sumerians were a highly organized people in almost every aspect of their public lives and endured frequent wars. Under these conditions, it is extremely unlikely that they would have overlooked the obvious need for their soldiers' medical care. In attempting to reconstruct the history of military medicine in the ancient world, the task before us is to assemble the evidence, glue it together carefully with the cement of inference, and in the end hope that it remains intact.

Notes

1. Fielding H. Garrison, *An Introduction to the History of Medicine* (London: W. B. Saunders, 1967), 19. See especially the section entitled "Identity of Forms of Ancient and Primitive Medicine," 17–24.
2. The relationship between longevity and the grace of the gods as perceived by ancient peoples is explored in Barnett, "Only the Bad Died Young," 155–59.
3. The tale of the preservation of Western medical knowledge as a result of the Muslim invasion of Spain in the Middle Ages is a fascinating story involving the Nestorian heresy of the fourth century CE. A historical account of this important event appears in this volume's chapter 11 on Islamic medicine.
4. The establishment of the famous Alexandrian medical school and library provided the primary locus for Greek and Egyptian physicians to come together, compare medical approaches, and develop new techniques. The school was established almost three hundred years after Herodotus wrote.
5. Aldea and Shaw, "Evolution of the Surgical Management," 561.
6. Guido Majno, *The Healing Hand: Man and Wound in the Ancient World* (Cambridge, MA: Harvard University Press, 1975), 28.
7. Ibid.
8. Ibid.
9. Gurdjian, "The Treatment of Penetrating Wounds," 157.
10. A. T. Olmstead, *The History of Assyria* (Chicago: University of Chicago Press, 1951), 64.
11. No less an authority than Hippocrates testified to the importance of war in the development of medicine when he advised his students that the best medical schools were to be found on the battlefield.
12. None of this is to say that military physicians were so practically oriented as to be incapable of innovation and making larger contributions to the medical field. Quite to the contrary. The world owes military physicians a great debt for their contributions to both science and medicine, as this book makes clear.
13. The U.S. Army posts its doctors for training to the Medical Shock Trauma Acute Resuscitation (MedSTAR) trauma center in Washington, D.C. The idea for a trauma center to deal with battle wounds encountered in civilian life was the brainchild of an English military physician.
14. Majno, *Healing Hand,* 59.

15. Garrison, *Introduction to the History of Medicine*, 54. It must be noted, however, that the splint appears on the body of a mummy.
16. Ibid., 62–63.
17. Ibid. The caduceus originated in Mesopotamia, where it was the symbol of Ningishzida, the god of fertility. To the Greeks, the caduceus was the emblem of Mercury and a symbol of commerce. The Romans used the same symbol as a sign of secrecy and neutrality, and peace envoys carried it. The association of the caduceus with peace led the U.S. Army Medical Corps to adopt it in the 1920s as the insignia for its branch of service.

3

ANCIENT SUMER, 4000–2000 BCE

Iraq is the site of ancient Sumer and Akkad, two city-states that produced the earliest armies of the Bronze Age. The Greeks called the area Mesopotamia, or literally "the land between the two rivers," a reference to the Tigris and Euphrates basin. In the Bible the area is called Schumer, which is the Sumerian word for the southern part of Iraq, or the site of Sumer and its capital city of Ur. About two hundred miles north of Ur is the site of ancient Akkad.[1] In 2300 BCE, Sargon the Great launched a campaign of conquest from Akkad that united all of Mesopotamia and gave the world its first military dictatorship.

Sumerian civilization was among the oldest urban civilizations on the planet. It was in Sumer that writing first emerged to produce ancient cuneiform, a form of record keeping written as wedged strokes on clay tablets, and that the first detailed records of military battles written or carved in stone appeared. In 4000 BCE, the cities of Sumer were the world's first examples of genuine urban centers of considerable size. One of these cities, Uruk, was enclosed by a wall 5.5 miles long.[2] According to information on the Tablets of Shuruppak (2600 BCE), a typical Sumerian city-state covered about 1,800 square miles, including all its lands and fields. This area could sustain a population of approximately thirty thousand to thirty-five thousand people. A population of this size could support an army of regular and reserve forces of between five thousand and six thousand soldiers at full mobilization.[3] The tablets record a force of between six hundred and seven hundred elite soldiers serving as the king's bodyguard, or the corps of the professional army.[4]

51

Sumerian society demonstrated a high degree of cooperative human effort that made urban life possible on a large scale. This cooperation was evident in the construction of dikes, walls, levees, irrigation canals, and temples, especially the giant ziggurats that date from the fourth millennium. An efficient agriculture freed large numbers of people from the land and allowed Sumer to develop a social order made up largely of freemen who met in concert to govern themselves.[5] The early Sumerian cities were characterized by a high degree of social and economic diversity that gave rise to artisans, merchants, priests, bureaucrats, road and temple architects, and professional soldiers.[6]

Ancient Sumerian civilization comprised a polyglot of ethnic peoples that lived in city-states and shared essentially the same culture. All city-states had the same political institutions, economic practices, religious beliefs and rituals, gods, legends, administrative language, and general way of life. Not surprising, they also developed the same military forms. Sumerian civilization was so culturally uniform that when Sargon of Akkad (2334 BCE), a Semitic prince from the north, conquered Sumer, his new subjects did not regard him as a foreigner. Sumer existed as a separate and distinct civilization from 4000 to 2004 BCE, when the Third Dynasty of Ur, which arose after two hundred years of Akkadian rule, was destroyed by the Amorites. By 1700 BCE, Babylonian influence was ascendant and lasted until the Assyrian state replaced it in 1200 BCE. It, in turn, was destroyed at the hands of the Medes in 642 BCE. Thus, the civilization that began with Sumer, migrated to Akkad, then moved to Babylon and eventually to Assyria can be seen as the continual development of the same civilization. This evolution was certainly true of its medical tradition as well.

Sumer was the most advanced and certainly the most organized civilization of the early ancient world. The invention of writing was only one of Sumer's legacies to world culture. The Sumerians were skilled chemists and mathematicians of an empirical and pragmatic sort. They invented the sexagesimal system of place notation that became the forerunner of the Hindu-Arabic decimal system in use today and introduced the world's first system of uniform weights and measures. They conceived the circle as having 360 degrees and invented the potter's wheel, the sailboat, and the first wheeled vehicles. The Sumerians were excellent architects and may have been the first to use the dome, the vault, and the arch.[7] They gave the myth of creation and the great flood to the world, stories that the Jews incorporated into the Bible during their Babylonian captivity and passed ultimately to the West.

Sumerian military medicine cannot be understood apart from the organizational development of the armies of the Sumerian city-states. The armies' high level of military sophistication was the result of more than a thousand years of warfare, which provided the impetus for a number of remarkable military innovations. The evidence for these innovations appears on the military monument from 2525 BCE known as the Stele of Vultures and in the surviving written records of the battle in which King Eannatum of Lagash defeated the king of Umma.[8]

The Stele of Vultures portrays Sumerian troops arranged as spear-bearing infantry fighting in a phalanx formation. The training required for this formation suggests the soldiers were professionals. As such, the monument provides the first evidence of a standing, professionally trained army.[9] The monument also displays for the first time soldiers wearing helmets. Excavation at the Death Pits of Ur confirms that the helmets were made of copper with a leather or woolen cap worn underneath.[10] The soldiers on the monument are equipped with cloaks upon which are sewn metal disks with raised spines, resembling the boss of a shield, in the first example of body armor in history. Later, the Sumerians invented plate armor made of bronze. The stele's lower palette shows the king holding a sickle-sword, a weapon that was a major innovation for its time and later became the primary weapon of Egyptian and Biblical armies. The stele also portrays the king riding in a chariot drawn by onagers, showing the first military use of the wheel.[11] It is clear from other sources that the Sumerians were the first to introduce a military veterinary corps staffed by "doctors of donkeys" and "doctors of mules."[12] Later archaeological evidence shows that the Sumerians were the first to develop the socketed ax, the deadly penetrating ax, and the composite bow—all major military innovations that greatly influenced the conduct of war for the next fifteen hundred years.[13]

The almost constant state of war in ancient Sumer influenced more than military technology. War shaped social and governing institutions as well. Priests ruled early Sumerian society, with warriors in a secondary role. By 2600 BCE, and perhaps earlier, a secular politico-military leadership displaced the priests in secular matters. The Tablets of Shuruppak show that at this early date, the kings of the city-states provided for the maintenance of six hundred to seven hundred soldiers on a full-time basis. The provision of military equipment for the soldiers was also a royal expense.[14] By 2400 BCE, the Sumerian kings had largely abandoned their religious functions while increasing their scope and control of secular functions.[15] The priests were excluded from secular matters beyond officiating at public ceremonies, and the king was no longer the high priest of the city, as he had been since ancient times, and no longer presided over religious festivals. His primary responsibility was to maintain and lead the army in defense of the city-state.

There is no reasonable way in which the city-states of ancient Sumer could have waged so much war and developed their innovative military technology without a high level of military organization to accomplish both. The organizational sophistication of Sumerian armies can be gauged from the surviving descriptions of the army of Sargon I, the first king to unite all the city-states of Sumer under a single ruler. In his fifty-year reign, he fought thirty-four wars, and his army of fifty-four hundred men was the largest standing army in the world at the time. The army was constructed around a corps of professional soldiers "who ate bread before the king" and was augmented by conscripts.[16] Sargon's army comprised nine battalions of six hundred men each that were commanded by a *gir.nita* (colonel). These battalions were divided into companies of sixty men each and were commanded by a *pa.pa/sha khattim* (company commander). Each company was subdivided into *nu.banda* (platoons) and platoons into *ugala* (squads), and these formations remained unchanged since ancient Sumerian times. Sargon's nobles were *niskum*, a class of soldiers who held plots of land awarded by the king in return for their military service. These feudal barons were used as a domestic police force to suppress rebellions.[17] Equipping an army the size of Sargon's required a high degree both of military organization to carry out its weapon and logistical functions and of routine administration, which was characteristic of a literate people who kept prodigious records.

While the evidence for Sumerian military organization is incomplete, it is not reasonable to expect that a people who tamed the violent Tigris and Euphrates Rivers with an elaborate system of dikes, canals, and bridges, and who sustained a sophisticated system of irrigation agriculture would have left to chance the organization of the military establishment upon which its society's survival depended. That the military protection of the state by the king—liter-

ally "the Big Man"—was regarded as the government's most important function suggests otherwise.

Sumerian Medicine

The Sumerians invented the first standards of medical ethical conduct. These
principles were later incorporated into the Babylonian Code of Hammurabi
as laws 215 through 223, which set statutory fees for physicians and penalties
for malpractice. These ethical precepts eventually made their way to the West,
where they were incorporated into Hippocrates's code for physicians. The
medical knowledge of the Sumerian period was highly empirical and pragmatic. It was only during the later Babylonian period of Sumerian-Babylonian-
Assyrian culture (1700–600 BCE) that it became corrupted by the rise of a
mystical numerology that was passed to the Jews as Kabbalah. Both traditions,
empirical and mystical, influenced later medical practice.

Attempting to describe the medicine of ancient Sumer is somewhat akin
to piecing together a portrait from a few random pages of an old medical book.
The information available to the historian is derived from two surviving clay
cuneiform tablets that served as medical texts, complemented by an analysis of
the Sumerian language and literature that contain a number of medical terms.
Separating the medical tradition of the Sumerian period (4000–2000 BCE)
is difficult because after 2000 BCE Sumerian civilization was eclipsed and
wholly incorporated into the Assyro-Babylonian civilization that lasted until
the sixth century BCE. This integration brought about a change in language
and written form. Fortunately, the ancient medical tradition of Sumer was
passed in toto and without interruption to Babylon and then to Assyria, where
it formed the spine of Assyro-Babylonian medicine. Literary analysts suggest
that the presence of Sumerian medical terms in the Babylonian and Assyrian
languages of the later period originated in the Sumerian period in much the
same way that Latin and Greek medical terms are still found in present-day
Western medical vocabularies even though some question whether the ancient
Greeks and Romans used the terms to mean the same thing that we have taken
them to mean. Thus, the separation of the medical traditions of the Sumerian and Assyro-Babylonian periods is somewhat artificial, while its continuity
provides the evidence for deducing the state of medical knowledge in ancient
Sumer.

Three types of physicians practiced Sumerian medicine in the third and fourth millennia BCE: the *Baru* (seer or sorcerer) who specialized in divinations and prognoses, the *Ashipu* (priest) who specialized in incantations and exorcisms, and the *Asu* (medical technician) who treated disease and injury with clinical techniques.[18] This division of medical practice among priests, sorcerers, and medical technicians more or less characterized the general practice of ancient medicine until the collapse of the Roman Empire. Even during the classical period in Greece when the scientific method was making progress, its impact was largely confined to a few physicians, while large segments of the population continued to rely on witchcraft and seers for medical treatment.[19]

The Sumerian physician occupied middle-class social status in Sumerian society and was very well educated by the standards of the time. He attended the *edubba* (general education school), where he learned to read and write the complex Sumerian language composed of hundreds of cuneiform signs and thousands of meanings. His medical education was obtained through lectures given by practicing physicians. These lectures were written on clay tablets, and the student was required to copy the lectures and other medical information repeatedly until he had committed them to memory. The Babylonians and Assyrians used the same system to train their physicians, so the medical knowledge of the prior period was easily preserved.[20]

The first physician noted in Sumerian records was "Lulu the doctor," whose name appears on a tablet found at Ur dating from 2700 BCE.[21] Another doctor, Urlugaledinna, appears on a seal of the twenty-fifth century BCE as a physician attendant to the king of Lagash.[22] This inscription is important, for it indicates that even at this early date the clinical medical practitioners had established their position around the king and eclipsed the influence of the medical priesthood in secular affairs. The Sumerians, like the Babylonians and Jews, required a doctor to prove himself competent in the medical arts through an apprentice program before he was allowed to practice. A physician who lost or injured too many patients could be fined by the state, sued by the patient, or have his license revoked. In Babylon, the state could even execute an incompetent physician who caused repeated harm. These professional, ethical, and legal codes demonstrate the seriousness with which the Sumerians regarded the practice of medicine.

Sumerian Military Medicine

At an early date, perhaps 2400 BCE, the Sumerian king relinquished his major religious functions and expanded his secular role, a development that relegated the once-powerful priesthood to secondary status. The result was that the Baru and Ashipu remained under the control and influence of the priesthood while the practitioners of clinical medicine, the Asu, came under the control and influence of the king. Separating empirical medical practice from the priesthood made it possible to develop a strong tradition of pragmatic medicine relatively free from theological and magical strictures. Moreover, the king, who was responsible for raising and maintaining the army and for protecting the state, then had an important resource to provide medical care for the army. The Asu was a member of the royal court and responsible directly to the king for the health of court members, including military personnel and their dependents.[23] It seems likely, then, that the Sumerian armies of the third millennium were the first armies in the world to provide medical care to their soldiers.

A surviving clay fragment contains a letter that records the difficulties that a commander stationed at a remote military post encountered. With the outpost under assault, the commander's letter to the king reads: "To my Lord say this: thus speaks Itur-Asdu, thy servant. There is no physician, no mason. The wall is crumbling, and there is no one to rebuild it. And if a sling-stone wounds a man, there is not a single physician. If it please my lord, may my lord send me a physician and a mason."[24] The letter implies that Sumerian military garrisons were accustomed to having medical support on station, and it is likely that military doctors were regularly posted to military garrisons.[25]

Given the information on the Tablets of Shuruppak mentioned earlier, it seems clear that physicians regularly attended the army in the field, or at least they did in the army of Lagash. Yet another surviving document details the complaints of some soldiers that the doctors remained in the rear of the battle because they were considered too valuable to risk being captured or killed. Taken together, the fragmentary evidence supports the conclusion that military physicians were present in the army of Sumer, accompanied the army into the field, and treated at least the king and senior officers in garrison and in the field.[26] The doctors' presence at remote garrisons suggests as well that some of these physicians were full-time military personnel rather than conscripted only in wartime. It is the first evidence of a military medical corps in the armies of the ancient world.

It is likely that the troops as well as the officers received medical care. Ancient Sumer was a relatively open society largely of freemen who governed themselves through a type of national councillor government. In the *Legend of Gilgamesh*, even the warrior king had to secure permission of the council to go to war. These freemen had rights that the king could not lightly ignore. It is unlikely that a society that maintained a core, standing professional army filled out by conscripts during times of war would not provide medical care when the means to do so were available. At the very least, medical care must have extended to the professionals.

Moreover, the army's care and maintenance were major responsibilities of the Sumerian kings whose city-states were at war with one another for a thousand years. Early documents (2700 BCE) make it clear that the king was responsible for housing, feeding, and equipping the army.[27] It is unlikely that this support would not have included medical care given its availability, if for no other reason that trained soldiers were expensive. It is also unlikely that any society that thought enough about medical practice to enact and enforce a code of medical ethics and behavior would not have extended the regulation of medical practice to the military physician as well.

The Stele of Vultures provides a glimpse into the physician's role in the Sumerian army. The stele shows the wounded of Eannatum's army being assembled in a single place after the battle. Why assemble them at all if not for examination and treatment? The stele also shows trenches being prepared for the dead of the victorious Sumerian army, while the enemy dead are left to be ripped apart and carried off by birds of prey and animals.[28] The organized burial of the dead and the assembly and treatment of the wounded remain two major functions of all military medical services to this day. There is no good reason to assume that they were not so in ancient Sumer.

How effective was the medical care available to the Sumerian soldier? As with all peoples of the early ancient period, disease was regarded as the work of demons that wrought their will on humankind. In a general sense, a belief in demons served the same function for the ancients as germ theory did for doctors of the modern age. For many years modern physicians asserted that a given disease was caused by a germ or virus that the medical profession had not yet discovered or could not prove existed. Just as the germ theory of later eras, the Sumerians' belief in demons did not prevent their doctors from looking for clinical signs of how a disease progressed, for how it spread, or for ways to prevent or cure it. Thus, Sumerian physicians developed clinical indicators of disease contagion. For example, they had precautions for protecting oneself from mosquitoes, and the ancient Mesopotamian god of disease and death was Nergal, who took the form of a fly.[29] It would appear that Sumerian doctors were aware of the insect vector as a factor in the spread of disease.

There is evidence, too, that the Sumerians had some notion of hygiene and contagion. Demons might cause disease, but people could take practical steps to avoid its onset and prevent transmission. In a surviving letter, a Sumerian physician demonstrates his remarkable understanding of the dynamics of contagion. The physician has given strict orders to the residents of a house containing a sick woman that "no one should drink in the cup where she drinks, . . . nor sit in the seat where she sits, . . . no one should sleep in the bed where she sleeps." The physician goes on to say that the woman should stop having visitors to the house because "this disease is contagious [*sabtu*, or "catching"]."[30] Here is the Sumerian physician at his best, unwilling to allow his own theoretical perspective that demons cause disease to interfere with his clinical experience.

The Sumerians, no less than the ancient trephiners of the eighth millennium BCE, believed that something could be done to prevent or cure illness. It is likely that since the causes of battle wounds were so obvious, the Sumerians concluded that battle wounds constituted a special category of injury that could be dealt with in a clinical manner. In this regard, it is worth recalling that of all the medical practitioners, the Asu had the lowest status, perhaps precisely because neither the injuries he dealt with nor the treatments he performed involved the magical or mystical.

The oldest surviving medical text in the world is written in Sumerian cuneiform and dates from 2300 BCE.[31] It is almost six hundred years older than the oldest surviving Egyptian medical document, the Kahun Papyrus, written in 1850 BCE, and predates the rise of Greek empirical medicine by two thousand years. As with the Egyptian text, the Sumerian tablet provides recipes for the Asu's concoction and application of a number of medical poultices. The style of the clinical medical tablet is similar to that used to record lectures and other medical notes in the education of Sumerian doctors.[32] Physicians copied texts for their use as medical manuals, ensuring that a large body of pragmatic medicine would develop over the centuries and be passed to the next generation. The resulting medical tradition persisted in an unbroken line from Sumer to Assyria from 4000 to 642 BCE, or a period of thirty-four hundred years, until it was lost with the final destruction of the Assyrian state in the sixth century BCE. By comparison, the Western medical tradition is still in its infancy.

The Sumerian tablet from 2300 BCE contains fifteen prescriptions divided into three classes according to the method of application. Eight prescriptions are for poultices that are to be applied externally, and three contain formulas for mixing medicines that are to be taken internally. The remaining four are somehow to be "arranged over" the patient in a manner that is not specified. They may be environmental remedies such as the burning of medicinal herbs or incense or, perhaps, conducting some sort of rite.[33] What is most instructive, however, is that none of the remedies show a trace of the magical and mystical elements of medical practice that characterized the medicine of the Baru and the Ashipu.[34] The prescriptions reveal a highly empirical, rational, and clinical attitude toward medicine, similar to what the early Sumerians demonstrated in their approach to chemistry and mathematics. If the text was a medical manual of a practicing physician, it must have had therapeutic value. A Sumerian physician's reputation was his livelihood, and it is unlikely that he would have risked it lightly.

A second tablet of the same period is also a prescription and reflects the same clinical approach. The prescription reads,

Having crushed turtle shell . . . , and having anointed the opening (of the sick organ, perhaps) with oil, you shall rub (with the crushed shell) the man lying prone (?). After rubbing with the crushed shell you shall rub (again) with fine beer; after rubbing with fine beer, you shall wash with water; after washing with water, you shall fill (the sick spot) with crushed fir wood. It is a (prescription) for someone afflicted by a disease in the *tun* and the *nu*.

These two words describe the sexual organs, and it is possible that the prescription may be the world's oldest treatment for venereal disease.[35]

The evidence concerning the Sumerian physician's level of skill is fragmentary. Strong written and archaeological evidence shows that the *naglabu* (bronze surgeon's knife) was in use by 2500 BCE.[36] Given that the Neolithic period has presented a number of examples of surgical saws, and that trephining was practiced even earlier, the presence of the surgeon's knife is not surprising. One fragment seems to indicate that Sumerian surgeons may have gone so far as to cut into the chest cavity.[37] If Sumerian physicians actually attempted to open the chest cavity, then their level of surgical skill was very advanced indeed. What is clearer, however, is that Sumerian doctors knew how to locate and drain internal abscesses in the body and in the skull.

While Sumerian physicians had no empirical concept of what caused infection, they were thoroughly familiar with infected wounds. The Sumerians called infection *ummu* (the hot thing). The cuneiform symbol for inflammation was a hot brazier pot, and it was often portrayed as centrally placed within the body, quite apart from the wound itself, indicating that Sumerian doctors were familiar with fever as a generalized indication of illness.[38] The wound might be infected, but it was the body itself that was sick. The Sumerian medical vocabulary contained several words for fever, with other fever-like conditions localized on the skin or in other areas of the body having separate words. The Sumerian physician seems to have had an adequate medical vocabulary at his disposal for defining some clinical conditions.

Although Sumerian doctors were familiar with pus as a product of infection, there is no evidence that they developed any theories about good and bad pus, as were found later in Greek and Roman medicine. This fact suggests that the Sumerians did not regard the production of pus as an inevitable and natural part of the healing process. This later idea led Greek and Roman doctors to provoke infection in a wound, even when none was present, in order to stimulate the presence of good pus, a classic example of allowing theory to overrule clinical observation. Undoubtedly Sumerian physicians were aware of the problems associated with infected wounds, and some of the poultices described in the oldest Sumerian text could have been used for treating these conditions. Standard clinical practice seems to have involved the ability to feel for the solidity of an abscess and then prescribing heat to make a firm abscess ripe for lancing.[39] Some of these procedures when used with poultices may have been effective in dealing with infected battle wounds.

The Asu was trained to perform the "Three Gestures" when administering medical treatment for wounds.[40] These protocols included washing the wound to cleanse it thoroughly, administering poultices, and bandaging the wound to hold the poultice in place. While the specific technique of loose bandaging per se is not mentioned and since suturing seems to have been unknown in Sumer at this time, bandaging a wound in a manner to hold a poultice in place would almost automatically result in a loose hold, allowing the wound to remain somewhat open and reducing the risk of anaerobic infection. Especially important was washing and cleansing the wound prior to bandaging, a technique that largely disappeared after the fall of Rome with horrifying results in military medical practice. The consequences of incomplete washing and tight and immediate bandaging produced enormous rates of tetanus and gangrene infections due to anaerobic bacteria.

The Sumerian military physician washed the wound with a mixture of beer and hot water, a treatment that modern medical authorities agree was excellent.[41] There is even some evidence from cuneiform texts and archaeology that Sumerian doctors used distillation pots to make chemical compounds. If so, they were the first medical practitioners to make distilled compounds for treating wounds or other ailments. Some of the earliest prescriptions in the Ur text call for heating a combination of resins, fats, and alkali, a procedure that would have produced a liquid soap for use as a wound washing agent.[42]

The Sumerians also developed an extensive *materia medica* (body of knowledge) of pharmacological compounds, many of which have been shown to be effective by modern standards.[43] Unlike the later Egyptian and Greek, Sumerian compounds were made largely from botanical sources.[44] Some of these botanical medicinals included extracts from thyme, mustard, plums, pears, figs, willow, manna, pine, *Atriplex halimus L* (Mediterranean saltbush), and *Prosopis stephaniana* (thorn plant).[45] The early doctors used common minerals, such as salt, river bitumen, and crude oil, which bubbled up from the ground in Mesopotamia.[46] The emphasis on botanical compounds is somewhat paradoxical in light of the fairly well-developed chemistry evident in Sumer at the time.

If one excludes simple distillation, the Egyptians seem to have been the first to use genuine chemical compounds for medical treatments, and they passed this emphasis to the Greeks. The root of the word *chemistry* in Greek is *chemi*, meaning "black." It is also the root for the Greek term for Egypt, which the Greeks regarded as the home of the "black arts" of chemistry and magic. Sumerian compounds made from plant extracts and resins were generally safer for wound treatment than the Egyptians' and Greeks' chemical salves and ointments, which often contained arsenic, mercury, and lead. Centuries of trial and error led the Sumerians to develop an extensive and safe materia medica.

Using these compounds in poultices may appear primitive to the modern eye, but this criticism overlooks the fact that the revolution in chemical pharmacology that produced synthetic drugs is relatively new, generally dating from the early 1950s. Before then, natural compounds were the staple of medical treatment in all countries. Even penicillin and morphine were first used as natural compounds. The use of medicinal poultices to treat injuries was a common medical practice in all the world's armies until the early twentieth century and in some cultures remains so. Some modern armies still prefer using natural compounds to synthetic compounds in treatment. Russian medics, for example, still carry extract of valeriana, a mild tranquilizer produced from a root, to treat psychiatric casualties on the battlefield.[47] During World War II, Russian doctors used a compound called fips, which was made from mineral mud and was found to be highly effective in treating burns.[48] Russian psychiatrists in World War II also used injections of the extract from the aloe plant, used mostly in the West as a treatment for sunburn and insect bites, as an effective treatment for edema and brain scarring in soldiers with head wounds.[49] Herbal medicines and animal extracts remain a mainstay of both civilian and military medical practice in China. Given the modern military physicians' continued successful use of botanical compounds, there is reason to expect that Sumerian doctors, with their two-thousand-year-old tradition of clinical experience with plant and resin compounds, were equally effective in discovering compounds that worked well for certain clinical conditions.

Only recently has the effectiveness of herbal and other compounds for medical treatment been explored systematically. In 1943 Oxford University undertook the first systematic search of plant compounds for medical use while developing ways to handle medical problems encountered in World War

II. The Oxford study found that of 166 families of plants, 28 were effective in combating *staphyloccocus aureau,* E. coli, or both. In 1959 a second study of 2,222 plant extracts showed that 1,362 had some antibiotic effect.[50] In 1974 the United States funded a similar survey in the hope of finding natural compounds that might be effective against cancer. The practical experience of the Chinese and Russian armies in the modern era with plant and herbal drugs suggests that the military physicians of ancient Sumer also may well have had at their disposal a number of these compounds that were effective in treating a range of medical conditions.

In assessing the Sumerians' contributions to military medicine, we must remember that we have only fragmentary evidence from which to construct a composite portrait of Sumerian military medical care. Nonetheless, it seems reasonable that the Sumerians were the first to separate the clinical practice of medicine from the control of the priesthood, a development that allowed the emergence of an independent system of pragmatic medicine free from the strictures of magic and ritual. The importance of this fact cannot be overstated. In countries like Egypt, where the priesthood remained dominant in medical matters, pragmatic medicine declined. In the Middle Ages the Catholic Church's control of medicine resulted in a retrogression in medical practice to almost pre–Bronze Age conditions. Its religious strictures slowed the progress of medical discovery considerably. Even today, if science is to progress, it must remain unhindered by a priori religious convictions.[51]

The Sumerians were the first to record their medical practices and findings in writing. Their method of training doctors at professional schools that required copying medical notes, texts, and lectures on clay tablets ensured that their two thousand years of trial and error would produce an effective, pragmatic, and permanent tradition of medicine that could be passed from generation to generation and even from culture to culture. Consequently, as early as 2000 BCE, the Sumerians had amassed a large clinical corpus of medical knowledge and practice that, while it lacked coherent theory, had the virtue of being effective.

Placing the practitioners of this empirical tradition directly under the king and permitting the more magical and mystical elements of the medical profession to remain under the priesthood made possible the emergence of the first military care for which we have any evidence. Although the details of the medical corps remain unknown, at the very least it seems certain that the Sumerians were the first to use military physicians whose special task was the care of military personnel. In this sense, it seems only fair to attribute to them the first attempt to tend to soldiers wounded on the battlefield.

Notes

1. The site of Akkad has not been located with certainty. The best guess is that it was near the modern town of Kish, a modern suburb of Baghdad, some two hundred miles north of Ur. On the problem of locating the site of Akkad, see Nissen, *The Early History of the Ancient Near East*, 167–68.

2. Ibid., 72.

3. Georges Roux, *Ancient Iraq* (New York: Penguin, 1986), 137. A good modern history of ancient Sumer is in Harriet Crawford's *Sumer and the Sumerians* (Cambridge, UK: Cambridge University Press, 1991.)

4. See Yadin, *The Art of Warfare in Biblical Lands*, 2:313–28, for a discussion of this point as it relates to the ability to mobilize populations in the defense of a siege.

5. Robert L. O'Connell, *Of Arms and Men: A History of War, Weapons, and Aggression* (New York: Oxford University Press, 1989), 35.

6. Khadduri, "Sumerian Civilization," 950.

7. Ibid.

8. For a photographic reproduction of the Stele of Vultures as well as an explanation of its significance for military history, see Yadin, *The Art of Warfare in Biblical Lands*, 1:135–36. For some cautions as to its use as a source document, see Nissen, *The Early History of the Ancient Near East*, 155–56.

9. O'Connell, *Of Arms and Men*, 35.

10. An explanation of the finds from the Death Pits of Ur can be found in Roux, *Ancient Iraq*, 129.

11. In terms of the wheel's impact on the fighting ability of armies, its use for logistics far surpassed its influence on the battlefield. By the time the chariot became an effective battlefield vehicle first under the Hyksos and then the Egyptians, it bore no resemblance to the early Sumerian prototype. In fact, the earliest chariots were not fighting vehicles at all but a means of transporting the nobility to the battlefield. See Gabriel and Metz, *From Sumer to Rome*, 75–79. It seems likely that the wheel was not invented by the Sumerians but probably acquired from the Indians. For more on the cultural contact of Sumer with the Hindu cultures, see Elisabeth Caspers, "Sumer, Coastal Arabia, and the Indus Valley in Protoliterate and Early Dynastic Eras: Supporting Evidence for a Cultural Linkage," *Journal of the Economic and Social History of the Orient* 22, no. 2 (May 1979), 42–49.

12. Samuel Noah Kramer, *The Sumerians: Their History, Culture, and Character* (Chicago: University of Chicago Press, 1963), 99.

13. Gabriel, *Empires at War*, 1:59–60. See also Gabriel and Metz, *From Sumer to Rome*, chapter 3, for an examination of the effectiveness and influence of the Sumerians' weapons innovations on warfare in the ancient world.

14. Roux, *Ancient Iraq*, 129.

15. An account of this separation and its implications is found in Nissen, *The Early History of the Ancient Near East*, 140. The first linguistic evidence of this separation is found during the Early Dynastic period. The term *ensi* is used to designate the priests, while the term *lugal* designates the secular leader in charge of military operations. In addition, the term for palace is now written as *e-gal* and is clearly differentiated from the term *e* used for temple.

16. Gabriel, *Empires at War*, 58.

17. Ibid.

18. Kramer, *The Sumerians*, 290–91.

19. McGrew, *Encyclopedia of Medicine*, 186–87.

20. Both the preservation and transmission of Sumerian medicine to Babylon and Assyria are evident in that the eight hundred clay cuneiform texts found in the library of Ashurbanipal that survived the great fire of 612 BCE contain medical conditions and descriptions using Sumerian words, although the Sumerian language had not been commonly used for almost thirteen hundred years.

21. Kramer, *The Sumerians*, 99.

22. Ibid.

23. P. B. Adamson, "The Military Surgeon: His Place in History," *Journal of the Royal Army Medical Corps* 128, no. 1 (1982): 43–44.

24. Majno, *Healing Hand*, 66.

25. Additional evidence for the presence of physicians in military garrisons is that a number of later Babylonian medical texts were discovered in the ruins of a military outpost.

26. Adamson, "The Military Surgeon," 44.

27. Roux, *Ancient Iraq*, 129.

28. See the photo in Yadin, *The Art of Warfare in Biblical Lands*, 1:135.

29. Garrison, *Notes on the History of Military Medicine*, 28.

30. Roux, *Ancient Iraq*, 342.

31. Martin Levey, "Some Objective Factors of Babylonian Medicine in Light of New Evidence," *Bulletin of the History of Medicine* 35 (January–February 1961): 65. See also Kramer, *The Sumerians*, 93.

32. Kramer, *The Sumerians*, 93–99.

33. Ibid., 96.

34. Ibid.

35. Ibid., 99.

36. Robert Biggs, "Medicine in Ancient Mesopotamia," *History of Science*, eds. A. C. Crombie and M. A. Hopkins (Cambridge, MA: Harvard University Press, 1969), 100. See also Majno, *Healing Hand*, 42.

37. Majno, *Healing Hand*, chapter 2, note 84. The evidence is not convincing that the operation described was performed on a live patient. Another possibility is that the surgeons were draining an internal chest abscess.

38. Ibid., 56.

39. Ibid., 59.

40. McGrew, *Encyclopedia of Medicine*, 187.

41. Majno, *Healing Hand*, 48.

42. Ibid., 50–51.

43. Ibid., 64.

44. Kramer, *The Sumerians*, 97.

45. Ibid.

46. Ibid.

47. Richard A. Gabriel, *Soviet Military Psychiatry* (Westport, CT: Greenwood, 1986), 68–70.

48. Ibid.

49. Ibid.

50. Majno, *Healing Hand*, 64.

51. The influence of religious groups in the United States convinced the George W. Bush administration to restrict stem cell research, demonstrating that religious beliefs continue to limit scientific research even today.

4

EGYPT,
3500–350 BCE

The climate and geography of Neolithic Egypt favored the development of a large-scale agricultural society. The soil deposited annually by the 678-mile-long Nile was so rich that farming with simple stone tools could produce sufficient food to support as many as 450 people per square mile.[1] Egypt had a population of almost one million people as early as 3000 BCE.[2] Unlike the city-states of Mesopotamia, where slavery was used to free manpower from the land for war and other tasks, the fertility of the Nile Valley made slavery unnecessary, and Egyptian society was made up largely of tenant farmers and craftsmen.

The cultural development of Egypt differed from the Mesopotamian city-states in another important respect. Egypt's geography isolated the country from regular contact with the other states of the ancient world for almost three thousand years. The Mediterranean Sea to the north, deserts to the east and west, and mountains and the Nile cataracts to the south ensured that Egypt remained relatively cut off from the cultural, military, and medical developments occurring elsewhere in the Middle East. Until the seventeenth century BCE, when the Hyksos invaded, Egyptian medical and military development had been completely indigenous for more than two millennia.

Egyptian society of the fourth millennium was organized around province-like political entities called *nomos* that were ruled by individual *nomarchs* (chiefs). Over time, these nomarchs coalesced around two loose feudal kingdoms, Upper and Lower Egypt. In 3200 BCE, the king of Upper Egypt—known to history by the various names of Narmer, Menses, or, probably most correctly, Hor-Aha (The Fighting Hawk)—unified the two kingdoms by force.[3] He established his capital at Memphis and began the reign of the pharaohs of the Predynastic Period over a national state that lasted seven hundred years.

The kings who followed from 3100 to 2000 BCE expanded the Egyptian state. During this period a state bureaucracy came into existence, writing emerged as a tool of centralized administration, and the early political institutions were transformed into a highly organized theocratic state led by a divine pharaoh and supported by structured religious, administrative, and military institutions. The Egyptian army consisted of a small standing force of several thousand regulars and was augmented by militia forces that the nomarchs called to national service when needed. Egypt also introduced conscription in this period, levying one man in a hundred to military service each year. For the first time, there is evidence of distinct military titles and ranks. The size of the army remains unknown, but a number of fortresses built around 2200 BCE would have each required up to three thousand men per garrison, suggesting a total force of at least sixty thousand men.[4]

The armies of Egypt became more structurally sophisticated and organized over the next five hundred years. In the seventeenth century BCE, the Hyksos, a Canaanite people from the east, overran Egypt and occupied the country for 108 years.[5] The occupation introduced the Egyptian military to the most advanced weaponry of the day. The Egyptians acquired the helmet, bronze body armor, the chariot, composite bow, penetrating ax, and sickle-sword from the Hyksos. By the fifteenth century BCE, the Theban princes succeeded in driving out the occupiers. With a larger and better-equipped army, the pharaohs of the Eighteenth Dynasty—Amenhotep I (1546–1515 BCE), Thutmose I (1515–1512 BCE), Thutmose II (1512–1504 BCE), and Thutmose III (1504–1450 BCE)—forged an Egyptian empire that ruled the region from Lebanon in the north to Nubia in the south for the next five hundred years.

These imperial wars brought about significant changes in Egyptian society. For the first time, a truly professional military caste came into being.[6] The army became a genuine national force supported by national conscription with a levy of one man in every ten called to military service. The military structure shows signs of even stronger organizational articulation, with a proliferation of military titles and a clearer staff organization. Later, Ramses II organized the empire into thirty-four military districts to facilitate the army's conscription, training, and supply. Military units were reformed into combined arms divisions with a clear command and staff structure. With the introduction of the oxcart and the chariot, the Egyptians developed an effective logistics capability. Thutmose III developed Egypt's first national seagoing navy and carried out the first amphibious operations in history, against Canaan and Lebanon.[7] The Egyptian army of this period showed the same organizational sophistication evident in almost every other area of Egyptian society, including the medical profession.[8]

Some idea of the degree of centralized organization in Egypt can be obtained by noting that the Great Pyramids, begun in 2613 BCE by Snefru, were not built by slaves but by free farmers and peasants under military direction. The central administration of Egypt was able to require public works labor from a workforce of eighty-five thousand men to quarry and transport 2.3 million stone blocks, each weighing five tons, and to maintain the effort for twenty years. By carefully scheduling the work during the annual flooding, when farmers could not work the land and large stone blocks could be easily floated over flooded areas, the pharaohs built these great structures without disrupting the economy.[9] Almost every aspect of Egyptian life was highly organized and regulated, meanwhile, including religion and medicine.

The Sumerians' early separation of medicine from the dominance of religion never occurred in Egypt. Given the theocratic nature of the Egyptian state, which was ruled by a pharaoh believed to be divine, it is not surprising that medical practice remained in the grip of a religious caste that controlled every aspect of its development and practice. The priest-physicians originally served as mediators between the patient and Sekhmet, the goddess of disease and illness and used incantations, ceremonies, and sacrifices to cure illness. Over time, however, some priests acquired practical medical skills as a consequence of clinical observation and experience. These priest-physicians were known as *w'bw* (pronounced Wa'bau) and were priests first and doctors second. They practiced medicine in the temples and controlled the medical profession through their influence with the king.[10]

Egyptian medicine demonstrated a high degree of specialization, which the practices of the medical professionals fostered. The Egyptian doctor concentrated on only one disease or a small group of related diseases in a system similar to that of modern physicians and their own practice of specialized medicine. Writing in the fifth century BCE, Herodotus noted that in Egypt "the art of medicine is thus divided among them: Each physician applies himself to one disease only, and not more. All places abound in physicians; some physicians are for the eyes, others for the head, others for the teeth, others for the intestines, and others for internal disorders."[11] Although specialization had characterized Egyptian medical practice for centuries, it appears to have been more prevalent in Herodotus's day than it had been earlier.

Centralized religious control and medical specialization account for the general decline in the quality of Egyptian medicine discernible from 2000 BCE to the third century BCE. Earlier Egyptian medicine had developed a strong clinical emphasis, similar to that in Sumer, and was actually much more effective. It was only as the Egyptian state became increasingly organized and centered around religious functions that Egyptian clinical medicine began to weaken. By Herodotus's time, Egyptian medicine as a clinical discipline had reached its lowest ebb while the priests, whose livelihood and influence depended on their ability to explain and treat illness and disease through religion and magic, accumulated more power.

Paradoxically, the Egyptians' penchant for writing and recording important events and information promoted the dependence of their medicine upon religion. The priests controlled the medical schools, and their written texts used to train physicians incorporated the dominant religious view of medical theory and practice. Medical training and practice were conducted in strict conformity with these texts, the most important of which was the *Embre,* itself regarded as a sacred text. If an Egyptian doctor treated a patient according to the instructions of the book and the patient died, he was absolved of any negligence or penalty. If he deviated from the prescribed treatment and the patient died, however, the physician could be put to death.[12] Under these conditions, it is hardly surprising that medical practice remained under the control of the priesthood and that clinical medicine declined as the power of the priesthood increased over the centuries.[13]

At the same time, however, Egyptian medicine was regarded as high science, and the profession certainly must have attracted the best minds in the country. What military skill was to Sumer and mathematical astronomy to Babylonia, medicine was to Egypt even though its medical science grew increasingly theoretical and speculative. This static phase lasted almost a thousand years, until the Alexandrian conquest of Egypt brought Egyptian medicine into contact with Greek empiricism.

The transformation of the Egyptian medical profession into a quasi-secular religious cult, however, did not prevent the continuation of pragmatic medicine altogether. As with most cults, the medical profession was concerned with larger questions of faith and the connection between theology and disease. A range of medical practice dealing with injuries and conditions whose causes were clear, such as battle wounds, were not considered important enough for the priest-physician's ministrations. There persisted an entire class of medical practitioners who dealt with the more mundane medical conditions of the day in a clinical manner. The result was the development of a rich and effective tradition of pragmatic medicine that was left mostly unregulated and ignored by the Egyptian medical priesthood. These clinical practitioners were often found in the army.

Egyptian Military Medicine

While the priest-physicians treated the higher social orders, the practitioners of Egyptian clinical medicine were lower-status physicians called *swnw* (pronounced soo-noo).[14] The swnw were paid state employees assigned to serve on building sites, at burial grounds, or with the army.[15] Although they lacked social status, these practitioners were the true heirs to the tradition of clinical medicine that had begun three thousand years before the arrival of Alexander. Because they could write and were required to keep records, they produced a large corpus of pragmatic medicine that was available to soldiers and the lower orders of society. The swnw served primarily as attendants to the army in garrison and in the field and were highly skilled in dealing with wounds and injuries.

Egyptian empirical medicine has a long history, probably beginning around 3000 BCE. Archaeologists have uncovered a number of medical papyri that document its development. The first Egyptian physician for which we have evidence is Hesy Re, the Chief Doctor of the Teeth (dentist), who attended the pyramid builders of the Third Dynasty (2600 BCE).[16] The early dentists' level of skill is clearly shown in archaeological finds that reveal the first use of retentive prostheses, that is, bridges for teeth.[17] A mandible discovered at Gizeh dating to 2750 BCE shows two artificial holes drilled by some ancient dentist to drain an abscess of the jaw under the first molar.[18] Even at this early date, Egyptian empirical medicine was far advanced indeed.

An interesting aspect of early Egyptian clinical medical literature is that it is replete with examples of treating battle wounds. Although the Sumerians were frequently at war and had medical personnel with their armies, their medical literature, at least that portion that has survived, does not mention treating battle wounds. The frequent mentions of battle wounds in the Egyptian literature point strongly to a medical presence on the battlefield and a serious concern with treating battle-related injuries. Thus, for example, the Egyptians seem to have been the first to use the splint for treating fractures. Carvings on a doorpost of a physician's tomb in Memphis dating from 2750 BCE show the procedure for setting fractured bones.[19] The Egyptians also appear to have been the first to stiffen the splint by impregnating linen wrappings with gums and resins. The evidence for this dates to almost 2600 BCE and represents a major medical advance in the treatment of fractures. The ability to use semiflexible splints allowed the natural contour of the limb to be followed more closely as the bone healed, contributing greatly to a successful clinical outcome.[20]

The same door engravings represent what may be the earliest records of successful clinical surgery. These lintel hieroglyphics show surgeons performing a circumcision and operations on the neck (probably lancing a boil), extremities, and the knee.[21] There is no evidence that Egyptian physicians ever actually opened the chest cavity, something that may have occurred in Sumer. It is likely that the Egyptians' worship of the dead, a process controlled by the priest-physicians, may have militated against dissection and surgery. These strictures also would help explain the poor knowledge of anatomy evident in Egyptian medical texts.

As an interesting aside on the subject of surgery, early surgical knives were made from iron gathered from fallen meteorites.[22] The use of such expensive and rare instruments would have been restricted to the most wealthy and powerful priest-physicians. The more common field practitioner used lancets of copper and, later, bronze. There is evidence that these clinicians also made use of the first disposable scalpels fashioned from sharpened reeds.[23] By 2400 BCE, Egyptian doctors routinely practiced surgery on the body. Recently discovered remains in what appears to be a military graveyard dating from that time reveal the routine use of splints and bandages and contain the world's oldest bloodstains.

Named after its discoverer, the famous pathologist G. Elliot Smith, the Smith Papyrus is among the most important evidence of Egyptian clinical practice. Dated as having been written around 1600 BCE, it is a scribe's copy of a medical text that was first compiled between 2600 and 2200 BCE. Medical texts were common because the medical schools and temples published and sold them to physicians and students to ensure consistent medical information and practice, or the same reasons why medical texts are used today. The Smith Papyrus appears to be the medical manual of a military surgeon.[24] The text is an almost complete manual explaining the examination, diagnosis, and treatment protocols for forty-eight clinical surgical cases, most of which are typically for battle wounds.[25] While there are some incantations and spells, the information in the Smith Papyrus is overwhelmingly empirical in nature and treatment and what we would expect to find in a military medical manual used by the swnw.

The text reveals a level of clinical practice drawn directly from the physician's experience with battle wounds. It shows that the Egyptians understood the concept of generalized fever as an indicator of illness and had knowledge of the pulse as well.[26] Of the text's twenty-seven examples of head injuries for which there are diagnoses and protocols of treatment, most are of the type commonly received in war. One example is the treatment for dealing with depressed fractures of the skull, a common head injury in the Egyptian army, which did not use the helmet until the seventeenth century BCE. Egyptian doctors developed a modern technique for exploring the dura while feeling for a pulse on the brain. The text shows how to put pressure on the brain to produce involuntary body movements. It also describes how to lift the depressed bone fragments off the dura and to hold the skull bone in place with sophisticated bandages. The papyrus cautions the physician against mistaking a nondepressed fracture for a depressed fracture, advice still found in modern textbooks.

The Smith Papyrus also prescribes treatment for sword gashes to the skull and for typical injuries caused by the mace, the basic weapon of the Egyptian army at this time, to the nose, lower jaw, and temporal bone. It includes a detailed examination of the diagnosis and treatment of crushed chests, broken backs, crushed vertebrae, and the paralysis that often accompanies these injuries. Those soldiers involved in siege operations typically received crush injuries, which were also common among quarry and construction workers who built temples, forts, and monuments. Evidence from archaeology corroborates the military nature of the wounds. Two graveyards, both dating from 2000 BCE, contain the remains of fifty-nine and sixty soldiers, respectively. In one graveyard, forty-nine bodies show evidence of head and body wounds from mace blows and injuries from stones thrown from walls, and they are similar to those described in the Smith Papyrus.[27] The remains of sixty Egyptian soldiers who suffered a wider range of injuries, including gaping cuts and mace and arrow wounds, are found in the other graveyard.[28] Again the wounds are typical of those described in the papyrus. Whoever he was, the author of the Smith Papyrus was thoroughly familiar with the wounds that Egyptian soldiers were likely to suffer on the battlefield.

In 1907 another pathologist F. Wood Jones joined G. Elliot Smith and undertook the first paleopathological study in Egypt.[29] Among their conclusions was the observation that the most common fractures in Egypt of the second millennium were "probably caused by fending off blows at the skull with the mace."[30] Their data testify to the regularity with which soldiers suffered these types of injuries and, thus, the familiarity of military doctors with the resulting wounds. The rate of fractures among nonmilitary populations was much lower. A survey of six thousand Egyptian skeletons revealed that only one of every thirty-two individuals suffered a broken bone in their lives, or only 3 percent.[31] The degree of attention paid to broken bones in Egyptian medical literature, and the relatively low rate of broken bones that a doctor would likely have encountered among the civilian population, suggests that much of the clinical literature on the subject was developed through wartime experience.

Egyptian military physicians placed great emphasis on pragmatic medicine. This focus is evident in the treatment they developed for a gaping head fracture where the dura was not penetrated. In cases of depressed or comminuted fractures, the initial laceration was extended, with the skull surgically opened by cross-incision. Free fragments of bone were removed, and the wound was dressed with lint (probably tiny pieces of linen) soaked in warm wine and oil of rose and placed against the dura. Linen balls soaked in vinegar and oil of rose were then applied externally, and the wound allowed to drain by strips of silk and hemp. The head was then bandaged over with a dressing.[32]

In 1536 CE, the famous French battle surgeon Ambroise Paré used almost the same technique. Routine medical practice of the sixteenth century mandated that injuries should be cauterized with boiling elder oil. Paré once ran out of elder oil at the height of a battle. With no alternative to common practice, Paré dressed his soldiers' wounds with lint smeared with egg yolk, rose oil, and turpentine. Paré recalls that he "could hardly sleep for continually thinking about the wounded men . . . I had not been able to cauterize." In the morning, Paré found that those men he had treated with the new technique "had very little pain . . . , no inflammation, no swelling, and that they passed a comfortable night." The experience convinced Paré never to use the cauterizing technique again.[33]

The Egyptians were also familiar with the concepts of inflammation and infection. The Egyptian term for infection is *srf* (pronounced seref) and, like its Sumerian counterpart, is derived from the hieroglyphic for a hot brazier.[34] The key to fighting infection was to prevent its onset, and a number of clinical techniques outlined in the Smith Papyrus considerably reduced the risk of infection to the wounded soldier. One protocol instructs the physician to "draw the wound together with *ydr*," a word that translates as "stitches."[35] If the translation is correct, then the Smith Papyrus records the first known *medical* use of suturing. The first *archaeological* evidence of suturing on a human is found on a mummy dating from 1100 BCE, five hundred years after the transcription of the Smith Papyrus.[36] Another linguistic analysis of the papyrus suggests that ydr was not a suture but a clamp that used a combination of thorns placed through the lips of the wound and then was bound with string to hold the wound closed.[37] In either case, this technique would have been successful in reducing the onset of infection because it would have closed the wound relatively loosely and allowed it to drain and expel any foreign matter missed in the initial washing of the wound. If Egyptian military doctors used this technique with any consistency, it is probable that the wounded Egyptian soldiers suffered considerably lower rates of wound infection than those endured by armies until World War I, when rapid and tight closure of the wound was routine practice.

The Smith Papyrus records yet another Egyptian medical innovation for treating battle wounds without provoking infection, adhesive bandages. Probably made of strips of linen cloth or woven papyrus held together with resin from the gum of the acacia tree,[38] adhesive tapes are much better than sutures for preventing infection. They hold the margins of the wound in the right position without barring the exit of pus, and they spare the tissues the presence of a foreign body—a thread or a clamp—that might favor infection.[39] The effectiveness of adhesive bandages is supported by their reappearance in the nineteenth century, when the problem of wound infection was so great that it threatened to eliminate the use of surgery altogether.[40] Egyptian physicians probably obtained the idea for the adhesive bandage from Egyptian morticians who, Herodotus recorded, used gum and other adhesives to fasten linen wrappings to mummies.[41]

The first step in preventing wound infection was to clean it carefully and thoroughly prior to administering further treatment. As in ancient Sumer, the technique of washing wounds was apparently a routine part of Egyptian military medical practice. Egyptian physicians used washing solutions made from Fuller's earth, pounded lupines, and natural soda. All of them are mild astringents and antiseptics and would have worked well as wound washes.[42]

Curiously, the Smith Papyrus is silent on the subject of bleeding. It is inconceivable, however, that Egyptian battle doctors were unaware of this important element of medical treatment given the nature of the wounds they frequently had to treat. The earliest Egyptian medical document that mentions bleeding and how to deal with it is the Ebers Papyrus, written a century or so later than the Smith Papyrus. The Ebers protocol describes how a physician should use a red-hot knife to cut into a wound so that the heat from the knife will prevent bleeding as the wound is incised. Egyptian physicians were the first in history to employ hemostasis to minimize bleeding.[43] Greek and Roman physicians later used cautery, and it remained the primary method to stop surgical bleeding until the nineteenth century.

The ability to stop bleeding is perhaps the most crucial aspect of battlefield medicine. If major blood loss can be prevented, the soldier has much less chance of going into shock, which is the leading cause of death on the battlefield. There is no evidence that the Egyptians used the tourniquet, and the discussions of cautery and bleeding contained in the Ebers Papyrus appear

Figure 1. *Hieroglyphic text from the Ebers Papyrus describing the use of the hot knife for cautery*

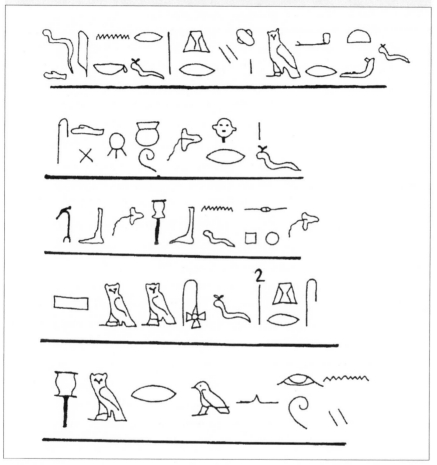

Figure by Tara Badessa

to be confined to surgical bleeding. There are, however, frequent injunctions in the Ebers document cautioning the physician against striking a blood vessel when using the knife. To stop bleeding in surgical procedures, the Egyptians placed small bits of crushed meat in the wound, a technique that introduced tissue enzymes and thromboplastins into the wound.[44] Modern medicine has long used this technique as an effective way to speed up clotting, and surgeons commonly used it to stem bleeding in the brain during surgical procedures as late as the 1940s.[45]

The extensive Egyptian materia medica comprised seven hundred identifiable plant and chemical compounds.[46] Among the most interesting of these botanical compounds was the extract of the poppy (opium), which was used early on as a soporific. By 1500 BCE, the Egyptians were regularly importing large quantities of distilled opium from Cyprus, and it is the first historical evidence for a drug used specifically as a painkiller or, perhaps, even a twilight anesthetic. Egyptian physicians also used salsalate, a compound similar to aspirin but without the risks of stomach bleeding. It is a powerful anti-inflammatory and painkiller that modern physicians still use to treat arthritis pain.[47]

The place of anesthesia in ancient medicine is puzzling. The term itself is modern. Oliver Wendell Holmes suggested using the Greek word *anaesthesia*, meaning "lack of sensation," to describe the effects of ether, the first effective modern anesthetic that military physicians started using in 1846.[48] Until then, as we shall see, every ancient medical tradition attempted to discover some method of relieving the pain associated with surgery. Moreover, some surgical procedures described in the ancient texts could not have been accomplished without some means of reducing, if not eliminating, the accompanying pain, and undoubtedly surgery without some form of anesthesia often risked the patient's death by shock. Yet, there are no discussions of surgical anesthetics per se in the surviving texts.[49] Because we now know that some of the compounds mentioned in the texts can be transformed into anesthetics, we are left to infer that ancient physicians *may* have used them in this manner, although we have no hard evidence that they did. But if these compounds were not used, then how were the surgeries described in the texts successfully accomplished? We simply don't know. We can be certain, however, that the search for a way to reduce the pain associated with surgery began early in recorded human history.

Egyptian physicians seem to have been fascinated with developing chemical compounds for medicinal uses. They commonly used copper salts, such as verdigris, malachite, and copper sulfate, in concocting new treatments. These "green pigments," as they were called, may have been used primarily for treating eye disease, a common scourge of Middle East peoples to this day. The green pigments became popular prophylactics for preventing eye diseases, and thousands of portraits of the period depict men and women wearing them as eye shadow.[50] When modern pathologists tested these salts they found them to be effective bacteriostatics against the types of bacteria often found in infected wounds. Some of these salts are still used today to treat staphylococcus infections, particularly impetigo.

By far the most common and effective wound treatment that Egyptian military doctors used was wild honey. Honey is mentioned in the Egyptian medical literature no fewer than five hundred times, and it was the main component in more than nine hundred medical remedies.[51] Modern biochemists conducted tests on the medicinal properties of honey and found it to be an excellent bacteriostatic and bactericide. When tested against seven types of common pathogenic wound bacteria, honey was found to kill these bacteria in less than two days on average and in some cases in less than ten hours—or rates equal to those achieved by modern antibiotics.[52] When mixed with salt, another common mineral compound used in Egyptian medicines, the bactericidal effect of these compounds increased significantly. In using honey to treat wound infections, the Egyptians had stumbled upon the most effective bacteria-killing compound available to physicians until the discovery of penicillin.

Honey also makes an excellent wound dressing because it is hypotonic and draws water from bacterial cells, causing them to die and preventing further reproduction. Moreover, honey contains glucose oxidase, an enzyme secreted by the bee's pharyngeal gland that is a powerful natural disinfectant and mild antibiotic.[53] Honey also contains propolis, a powerful bacteriostatic that prevents the spread of infection. When used with adhesive bandages and the loose closure of wounds, honey is an effective wound dressing. Adhesive bandages allowed the wound sufficient opening to drain, while the honey acted as a powerful draw to pull whatever pus or decayed matter had been left in or had infiltrated the wound. At the same time, honey exercised a strong bactericidal effect to prevent the development of further infection.

Another Egyptian wound dressing used onion and garlic oil and paste. Both of these botanical compounds are more effective against gram-negative bacteria than is penicillin. These pastes and oils were most beneficial in fighting wounds to the stomach or intestines, which usually became infected from gram-negative bacteria in the gut.[54] In yet another treatment for infection, public works crews in Egypt were fed large quantities of radishes to ward off illness and infection.[55] Biochemists have isolated a substance called raphanin from an extract of radish seeds that is an effective antibiotic against a number of bacteria, including *cocci* and coli.[56]

Clearly Egyptian physicians developed numerous medical compounds and clinical practices that worked well in treating battle wounds. Far less clear, however, is the structure of the Egyptian military medical service itself. No surviving evidence tells how the medical service worked, how it was staffed, or who directed it. What follows, therefore, is a portrait of the Egyptian military medical service pieced together largely from fragmentary data and inference.

It seems safe to assume that given the influence of the priest-physicians and the worship of the dead as major elements in Egyptian society that priests were important and powerful figures at the Egyptian court. As such, it is likely that these physicians accompanied at least the king and his senior generals, who were often members of the pharaoh's extended family, when on campaign. The pharaohs were also field commanders and usually went with their armies into the field. It is unlikely that they would have ventured forth without some provision for their own medical care. This pattern of the leadership employing personal physicians was common in Sumer and Greece as well.

It seems likely that the common soldier also had some medical resources at his disposal. One source notes that "on campaigns or other expeditions out of the country, the sick are treated without cost to themselves; for the physicians receive compensation from the state."[57] This observation seems to imply that clinical medical practitioners, or the swnw, regularly accompanied the army. The state employed these same clinical practitioners to provide medical care to the workers on public works projects, so it seems likely that an army as organized and sophisticated as the Egyptian army would have used the swnw to treat its military personnel as well. The Egyptian military required the use of defensive garrisons positioned at key points on the country's borders. A number of medical texts have been found in the remains of these forts, suggesting that it was common practice to post military physicians in them on a regular basis.

The empirical tradition of Egyptian medicine drew most of its clinical observations from those wounds and injuries commonly encountered in military life and on the battlefield. Archaeological evidence from Egyptian cemeteries confirms this theory. It does raise the question of who observed and described these clinical treatments if not military physicians. It is unlikely that the priest-physicians would have ventured into the tawdry business of field medical care on a regular basis. Moreover, since the nature of military injuries needed little explaining, it is possible that the clinical tradition developed outside the mystical medical tradition. This informal approach may account somewhat for the lack of descriptive evidence of a military medical service. As with other aspects of military life, it may have been regarded as too obvious to require the attention of the more "important" elements of the medical profession.

This analysis does little to remove the central mystery of Egyptian military medicine that, while no hard evidence of a military medical service in the Egyptian army has survived, the most commonly documented clinical conditions and treatment techniques are those developed to treat typical battle wounds. The lack of evidence for a formal military service remains a glaring omission in an army that organizationally had developed to almost modern standards. More puzzling is that as Egypt began its age of empire in the seventeenth century BCE, a period when its military was most active, Egyptian medicine began a long period of decline into magic and mysticism. Its practitioners shunned medicine's empirical aspects precisely at a time when the increased frequency of war provided more opportunities for clinical observation. By the time the Greeks conquered Egypt in the third century BCE, the quality of Egyptian medicine was at its lowest ebb. It was through the influence of Greek empirical physicians that the Egyptian tradition of pragmatic medicine received renewed stimulus and returned to its ancient clinical roots.

Notes

1. Wenke, *Patterns in Prehistory*, 468.
2. Ibid., 486.
3. Leonard Cottrell, *The Warrior Pharaohs* (New York: Putnam, 1969), 18–19.
4. Ibid., 51.
5. Gabriel, *Thutmose III*, 31. See also David O'Connor, "The Hyksos Period in Egypt," in *The Hyksos: New Historical and Archaeological Perspectives*, ed. Eliezer D. Oren (Philadelphia: University of Pennsylvania Press, 1997), 48.
6. Raymond W. Baker, "History of Egyptian Civilization," *Encyclopaedia Britannica*, 15th ed. (Chicago: Encyclopaedia Britannica, 1985), 148–62.
7. Richard A. Gabriel, "Amphibious Pharaoh," *Military History*, October–November 2009, 42–49.
8. Gabriel, *Thutmose III*, 83–87.
9. Gabriel, *Culture of War*, 36.

10. A. Rosalie David, *The Ancient Egyptians: Religious Beliefs and Practices* (London: Routledge and Kegan Paul, 1982), 141–43.

11. Garrison, *Introduction to the History of Medicine*, 57, quoting Herodotus, book 2, 84.

12. D. S. Gordon, "Penetrating Head Injuries," *Ulster Medical Journal* 57, no. 1 (April 1988), 2. These same draconian penalties are found in the Babylonian Code of Hammurabi. The prevalence of the legal theory of *lex talonis* found therein is somewhat puzzling in the case of the Hammurabi Code, which was clearly based upon earlier Sumerian prototypical codes of medical ethics. While fines and other civil penalties were levied upon Sumerian physicians found guilty of malpractice, there is no evidence that the offense ever carried the death penalty.

13. This same situation prevailed in Europe until the Reformation. Even then, the medical profession continued to instruct its practitioners in practices that were more heavily rooted in religion than in clinical experience. Although neither educated nor recognized by the profession as legitimate practitioners, the military doctors of this period developed a tradition of clinical medicine based on their battlefield experience.

14. David, *The Ancient Egyptians*, 142. See also Majno, *Healing Hand*, 69.

15. David, *The Ancient Egyptians*, 142.

16. Curt Proskauer, "A Pictorial History of Dentistry, Part I—Prehistoric, Egyptian, Assyrian," *TIC Journal* 38, no. 2 (February 1979): 8.

17. Ibid., 10.

18. Ibid.

19. For an analysis of these hieroglyphics and what they mean, see Bayard Holmes and P. Gad Kitterman, *Medicine in Ancient Egypt: The Hieratic Material* (Cincinnati: Lancet Clinic Press, 1914), 14. This work presents a complete description of the contents of the major Egyptian medical papyri and is a primary source of information on Egyptian medicine.

20. Dennis J. Callahan and Bernard J. Harris, "A Short History of Plaster-of-Paris Cast Immobilization," *Minnesota Medicine* 69 (April 1986): 195.

21. Holmes and Kitterman, *Medicine in Ancient Egypt*, 16.

22. This fascinating tale is taken from Majno, *Healing Hand*, 86–88. The hieroglyph for lancet is derived from the root Egyptian hieroglyph for star. The use of iron surgical knives fashioned from meteorites may have delayed the use of bronze knives for almost a thousand years, even though the technology for making bronze lancets was readily available.

23. Ibid., 90.

24. Norman Lester Rowe, "The History of the Treatment of Maxillo-Facial Trauma," *Annals of the Royal College of Surgeons* 49, no. 5 (1971): 330, for the claim that the papyrus may be a military medical manual.

25. Garrison, *Introduction to the History of Medicine*, 55.
26. Ibid. See also Holmes and Kitterman, *Medicine in Ancient Egypt*, 16. A more modern analysis of Egyptian medicine is found in John F. Nunn, *Ancient Egyptian Medicine* (Norman: University of Oklahoma Press, 1996).
27. Gurdjian, "The Treatment of Penetrating Wounds," 158.
28. Garrison, *Introduction to the History of Medicine*, 59.
29. *Archaeological Survey of Nubia*, Bulletins 1–7 (Cairo: Ministry of Finance, Survey Department, 1910). The data referenced here are found in volume 2.
30. Ibid.
31. Majno, *Healing Hand*, 84.
32. Gurdjian, "The Treatment of Penetrating Wounds," 158.
33. Charles G. H. West, "A Short History of the Management of Penetrating Missile Injuries of the Head," *Surgical Neurology* 16, no. 2 (August 1981): 146.
34. Majno, *Healing Hand*, 98–101.
35. Ibid., 91–92.
36. Ibid., 93.
37. Ibid.
38. Ibid., 94.
39. Ibid., quoting Herodotus.
40. Ibid., 96.
41. Ibid.
42. Rowe, "The History of the Treatment of Maxillo-Facial Trauma," 331.
43. Majno, *Healing Hand*, 105–7.
44. Ibid., 108.
45. Ibid., 111.
46. For an overview of the Egyptian pharmacopoeia and that of other ancient cultures, see Anna DePasquale, "Pharmacognosy: The Oldest Modern Science," *Journal of Ethnopharmacology* 11 (1984): 1–16.
47. *Boston Globe*, March 16, 2010, B-4.
48. American doctors during the Mexican War of 1846 were the first to use modern anesthesia.
49. Christine Salazar, *The Treatment of War Wounds in Graeco-Roman Antiquity* (Boston: Brill, 2000), 64. "Nowhere in the treatises dealing with surgery is there any mention of anesthesia."
50. The practice of surrounding the eye with a shadow of green pigment to ward off disease persists to this day in the region with people outlining the doors of houses with green paint to thwart sickness or bad luck.
51. Majno, *Healing Hand*, 116–17.
52. Ibid.
53. Ibid.

54. My thanks to Professor Tom Lee of the Biology Department at Saint Anselm College for his help in explaining the role of gram-negative bacteria in stomach and intestinal wounds.

55. The Jewish ceremony of Passover requires the eating of *maror*, or the bitter herb, to remind one of the days when the Israelites were in bondage in Egypt. This bitter herb is the radish, perhaps recalling when the Israelites were fed radishes while they were forced to work as corvée laborers on the pharaoh's "store cities" as noted in the Bible.

56. Garrison, *Notes on the History of Military Medicine*, 25.

57. Ibid., quoting Diodorus Siculus, book I, 82.

5

ASSYRIA,
911–612 BCE

The Assyrian Empire was the direct descendent of the earlier Sumerian civilization, a fact that had important implications for the Assyrians' practice of medicine. Historians refer to the period beginning with Hammurabi in the seventeenth century BCE and ending with the destruction of the Assyrian state in 612 BCE as the Assyro-Babylonian period, a term emphasizing the homogeneity and continuity of the Mesopotamian culture during that time. From the end of the Third Dynasty of Ur until the demise of the Assyrian state, two major forces shaped Mesopotamian culture: first, a period of foreign invasions by nomadic peoples who settled in the area and adopted the dominant Sumerian culture that had characterized most of Mesopotamia for almost two millennia and, second, attempts by the various states of the area to assert their power and regain control of the old Sumerian empire by force.

The Babylonian ascendancy lasted for 430 years, only to be replaced by a Kassite domination of foreigners that ruled for the next 400 years.[1] In the ninth century BCE after three hundred years of instability known as the Mesopotamian Dark Ages, Assyria, a traditional state of northern Mesopotamia, gained ascendancy and ruled over an area greater than the old Sumerian empire for three hundred years. During this Assyro-Babylonian period, the culture of the area remained essentially unchanged. The old Sumerian gods were still worshiped, cuneiform continued to be the official written language of the state, and artistic life and economic and medical practices remained basically the same.[2] The situation was not unlike the period after 400 CE when Europe, despite its non-Roman leadership and the settlement of the invading tribal populations, remained a world where Roman cultural institutions predominated and Latin was the official administrative language. Similarly, the Akkadian script that Sargon introduced to Sumer prior to 2000 BCE and written cuneiform continued to be used throughout the Assyro-Babylonian period until Aramaic and the use of the Phoenician alphabet replaced them in the eighth century BCE.[3]

Two significant changes affected the development of military medicine during this period: the Assyrian politico-military structure shifted, and the medical profession moved away from the three-thousand-year-old Sumerian model of practice. While Mesopotamia remained a nation of city-states, the political structure underwent a drastic transformation. The Assyrian kings had greatly increased the scope of their power over various aspects of civic life. All real power now rested with the throne. Assyria was totally reorganized along the lines of a military dictatorship, with the monarchy supported by a network of fully articulated bureaucratic institutions. A professional bureaucracy complete with written records and laws regulated most aspects of life. Supported by intelligence agencies and secret police to ensure order, military commanders governed the various provinces of the empire. The Assyrians imposed terror and cruelty upon their subject populations and employed their army as a primary tool of oppression. War was the national industry of Assyria, and it is not surprising that the Assyrians produced the largest, best-equipped, and most effective military machine the world had seen until that time. The strong degree of military centralization gave the army priority over all social resources, including the services of physicians. Assyria was the first state of the ancient world to establish a professional military medical corps.

The changes in the nature of the Assyrian medical profession are important in that they made it possible for an ancient army to have the first full-time military physicians. In the previous Sumerian civilization, medical practice had developed along dual lines of magic and empirical treatment, with the Asu being the primary practitioner of clinical medicine. This divergence is evident as early as 2500 BCE when the kings broke the power of the priesthood, kept the sorcerers and magicians under the tutelage of the temple, and put the clinical practitioners under the control of the king. This development resulted in the first regular use of physicians within the army, although the extent of their service is not certain.

This state of affairs remained essentially unchanged throughout the rise and fall of Babylon and the repeated invasions by tribal peoples until the beginning of the first millennium. During this period, physicians were still trained in schools, medical texts were copied, and medical knowledge increased, however slowly. During the period of Kassite rule (1595–1159 BCE), the medical profession changed as the status of the priest-physicians grew and that of the empirical practitioners declined.[4] This difference seems to have resulted from a general shift in religion that stressed resignation in the face of the gods instead of superstition over faith. It was marked by the appearance in medical literature of mystical numerologies, calendars of propitious signs, lists of demons, and increased collections of incantations.[5] It is unclear whether the priest-physicians took over the role of the Asu, but it is not likely since empiricism and magic were now at loggerheads. There was, however, a precipitous decline in the number of empirical texts copied, and the mentions of the Asu in civil correspondence greatly declined.[6] Thus, a strong spell of mysticism seems to have been cast over the medical profession, resulting in the empirical practitioner's loss of status. The importance of this development was that the Asu, deprived of status and independent income, became a government dependent; thus he could be called to practice his skills in military service.

Assyrian Medicine

The Assyrian penchant for keeping written records leaves us a good description of Assyrian medicine, and it is more complete than for any other period of ancient Mesopotamian history. An examination of these documents reveals the dual nature of Assyrian medicine and the high degree to which it was codified. Among the most important surviving records is the great number of medical texts discovered in the library of Ashurbanipal, king of Assyria from 668 to 626 BCE. His library ranks as one of the largest libraries of the ancient world and was not surpassed until the construction of the great library of Alexandria in the third century BCE. Assembled at Ashurbanipal's direction, the library contained more than 100,000 texts on various subjects. Thirty thousand of them survived the great fire that destroyed the library in 612 BCE when Assyria's capital, Nineveh, was crushed. Eight hundred medical texts survived in sufficient condition to be identified and translated.[7]

A subcollection of the library entitled *The Treatise of Medical Diagnosis and Prognosis* seems to have been copied around 1000 BCE.[8] It is a remarkable document and proves that the dual character of Sumerian medicine survived intact through the Assyrian period. The treatise presents three thousand medical case studies that offer accurate descriptions of numerous clinical conditions that physicians could expect to confront in their practice. Each set of diagnoses is followed by a set of recovery prognoses, concluding with the appropriate incantations and spells to use to ensure effective treatment.[9] Although the collection is really a set of texts meant to be used by priests and sorcerers and thus has a high concentration of magic in it, the diagnoses of the conditions described, if not the prescriptions, are so accurate that they could be based upon nothing else but clinical observation. Thus, the old Sumerian tripartite division of medical practice among the priest, the sorcerer, and the empirical practitioner is clearly evident.

This last point engenders some mystery insofar as the treatise reveals that the medical knowledge of the priest-physicians had taken on an empirical emphasis that was not present in earlier Sumerian medicine. The appearance of clinical elements in the magic literature of Assyrian medicine comes at a time when the priest-physicians had become even more mystical in their approach to medicine and when their power in Assyrian society was increasing. The concomitant decline of the Asu in social status, as far as can be determined, was not accompanied by the Asu's assimilation into the priesthood. The Asu seems to have remained a common and traditional feature of Assyrian society. The priest-physicians probably incorporated the clinical knowledge and practices of the Asu into their own literature as a way of demonstrating that they were familiar with it and to increase the general population's acceptance of them as effective practitioners. The priest-physicians, however, did not abandon their magical approach to medicine, and their clinical practice remained a subordinate activity. Perhaps the situation was akin to the relationship between chiropractors and the medical profession's physicians today.

The rise of mysticism during the Assyrian period did not result in the disappearance of the Asu or his practice of clinical medicine. Overwhelming evidence attests that the strong tradition of pragmatic medicine remained in practice. King Ashurbanipal testified in a surviving document that when he built his library collection, he attempted to incorporate the entire realm of medical knowledge available to the Assyrians.[10] Ashurbanipal noted on the commemorative tablet that he had registered in his library the three ways of healing: *pultitu* (the art of healing with drugs), *sipir bel imti* (the way of operating with the brass knife), and *urti mashmashe* (the healing that comes from the prescriptions of sorcerers).[11]

Additional evidence of the survival of the Asu and his pragmatic brand of medicine appears in other texts. Another set of texts, called the therapeutic texts, lists the symptoms and etiology of a number of diseases. These texts record various medical conditions, among them rumination (general stomach disorders), acid stomach, rheumatism, cardiac disease, and several liver and eye diseases. An additional number of well-defined clinical symptoms, including day and night blindness, paralytic stroke, falling sickness, scabies, and pediculosis, are easily recognizable to modern physicians.[12] The therapeutic texts seem to have been used to instruct the Asu in his clinical practice, and the references to demons and magical incantations contained within them are nominal.[13] There is also a letter dating from 1300 BCE in which the king of Babylon recorded that he had sent both a physician and a sorcerer to Muwatallis, the Hittite king, to cure the monarch's ills.[14]

By far the most important document showing the continuation of medical pragmatics in Assyria is an Akkadian medical text written in Hittite cuneiform. Both Hittite writing and medicine were direct imports from Babylonia, and the Hittites had no medical tradition of their own.[15] This clay tablet has writing on both sides. On one side is a completely clinical and objective prescript of a disease, while on the other side there appears a ritual for purification.[16] The tablet clearly demonstrates the parallel existence of the two Assyrian medical traditions.

What was the connection between these two traditions as they coexisted in practice? It seems certain that the Asu was never permitted to apply the major magical prescriptions. These processes were reserved to a priesthood jealous of its prerogatives in the same manner that priests today prohibit certain rituals from being practiced by laymen. It also seems unlikely that the priests would have become effective competitors to the Asu's daily practice, since there was little status, power, or money in doing so. Yet they must have had some connection, for both types of medical practitioners existed side by side for almost two thousand years.

Two linkages suggest themselves. First, the Assyrian materia medica was even more developed and extensive than that first found in ancient Sumer, a fact that testifies to some progress in clinical experimentation with drugs over many centuries. A document dating from the fourteenth century BCE records 250 drugs found on an apothecary's list.[17] While the use of these drugs could only have been medicinal, a great number of the Asu's drugs and compounds appeared for the first time in the priest-physicians' incantations and protocols.[18] Moreover, there appears to have been another connection. Assyrian physicians practiced extispicy, the art of divination by examining the internal body parts of animals.[19] Thus, they were familiar with the internal organs of animals and, through extrapolation, with those of the human body. The accuracy of these extrapolations remains unknown. But in at least one case concerning the anatomy of the human liver, their knowledge was extremely accurate.[20] While no hard evidence exists of any overt collaboration in medical studies between the two types of physicians, it seems likely that in a society in which both types of medical practitioners were literate and where copying medical texts was commonplace, the practical lessons learned by each type of physician were commonly shared.[21]

The general level of medical knowledge in Assyria was not, however, significantly better than what had existed in Sumer two millennia earlier. There had been some minor advances in the use of poultices and herbal compounds, but we have no evidence of any breakthroughs that would have made a great difference in a clinical sense. Surgery was still at about the same level as conducted in Sumer, and many of the references to surgical operations are also similar. The surgeon was competent to lance boils and abscesses and to perform simple operations to treat the eye diseases that seem to have afflicted the Assyrians as well as the ancient Sumerians.[22] The surgical instruments mentioned—the brass knife, spatulas, and tubes of metal to drain abscesses—appear rudimentary, and the Sumerians had employed them all two millennia earlier. Bandages were used, but there are no references to methods to stop bleeding as there are in Egyptian medical literature of this time.[23] That the Assyrians seem not to have practiced circumcision, trephining, or castration (eunuchs had their testicles crushed instead) might account to some extent for this lack of knowledge about bleeding. The level of empirical medicine in Assyria was probably little more effective than first aid.[24] Certainly the knowledge of infection and some poultices to prevent or "cure" infection would have been helpful to the military physician, but Assyrian field medicine was probably not as effective as that in Egypt.

The Assyrian army of the eighth century BCE was the largest and most sophisticated army of its time in terms of weaponry, tactics, siege craft, logistics, strategic and tactical mobility, logistical support and flexibility, and overall military efficiency. While later armies, notably those of the Persians and Alexandrian Greeks, surpassed the Assyrian army in some respects, no army equaled its overall organizational development and sophistication until the armies of Rome.

The Assyrian military establishment was thoroughly integrated into the larger social, political, religious, and economic institutions of the Assyrian state, and much of its success came from its ability to take maximum advantage of this affiliation. The primacy of the king as the nation's chief warrior led to the establishment of a political order that was in every sense a military dictatorship. The level of integration between the military and other social institutions of the Assyrian state was directed at the conduct of almost constant war.

Assyria emerged as the most powerful and successful military empire that the world had seen to that time, and its power was unabashedly built on military force and police terror. As in modern times, the constant threat of war created a war psychology that allowed the kings to extend their influence into all areas of Assyrian society and garner for the military whatever resources it required. Between 890 and 640 BCE, the height of Assyrian power, the Assyrians fought 108 major and minor wars, punitive expeditions, and significant military operations against neighboring states.[25] Sargon II (721–705 BCE) carried out 10 major wars of conquest or suppression in a mere sixteen years.[26] In the early days of the empire, Shalmaneser III (858–824 BCE) conducted 31 wars in his thirty-five-year reign.[27] Assyria became the largest military empire in the world of its day and had the largest, best-equipped, best-trained, and cruelest military organization the world had ever seen.

The far-flung and multinational Assyrian empire was not easy to govern with military force alone. To supplement military control, the Assyrians created a centralized and highly efficient bureaucracy to govern the empire on a day-to-day basis. This administrative apparatus was modern in every respect and reported directly to the king. The Assyrians instituted the imperial system of provincial management of conquered peoples, a system the Romans later adopted.[28] Military men often held high positions in the civil service and in conquered areas. Even in times of peace, the line between civil and military administration was often unclear.[29] As efficient as the administrative structure was, no Assyrian monarch was foolish enough to rely on it alone. Behind the civil service stood a police and intelligence apparatus operated by the king's personal bodyguard. These praetorians had the task of ensuring the loyalty of the civil servants and anyone in the country who might represent a threat to the royal will.[30] The bodyguard functioned as secret police, and the men employed the usual means to accomplish their task, including terminating officials who ran afoul of the king.

The high degree of organizational sophistication that characterized the Assyrian state was also evident in its military organization. Establishing and maintaining the empire required a military institution of great size. No accurate figures exist, but the army's size is estimated at between 150,000 and 200,000 men.[31] An Assyrian combat field army numbered 50,000 men with various mixes of infantry, chariots, and cavalry.[32] Even in the early days at the battle of Karkar (853 BCE), Shalmaneser III was able to put 62,000 infantry, 1,900 horse cavalry, 3,900 chariots, and 1,000 camels into the field against the Syrians. Shalmaneser records that at that battle "I slew 14,000 of their warriors. . . . The plain was too small to let their bodies fall, the wide countryside was used up in burying them."[33] The enemy strength was around 70,000 troops.[34]

The Assyrian army was the first genuine combined arms army of the ancient world, comprising infantry, cavalry, archers, chariots, siege specialists, siege engineers, tunnelers, scouts, sappers, and intelligence officers. Assyrian commanders were masters at utilizing these troops in combined arms operations.[35] The army was the first in history to be equipped completely with iron weapons, and their manufacture, storage, and repair were central features of the army's logistical base. A single weapons room in Sargon's palace at Dur-Sharrukin contained two hundred tons of iron weapons.[36] No army surpassed the organizational sophistication and skill of the Assyrians' military until the legions of Rome were formed.

Assyrian Military Medicine

The degree of social and military organization of the Assyrian state is an important element in understanding the role of the military physician that emerged during the Assyrian empire. Whatever the level of general medical knowledge in a society, the medical establishment cannot become a military resource unless the army that requires its use is also organizationally highly developed. Less organizationally developed military establishments, such as the armies of classical Greece, failed to utilize even their great amount of medical knowledge in a way that could make a difference on the battlefield. In Assyria, the pressure of constant wars against external threats, the centralization of authority in the warrior king, the organizational development of the army, and the changing social role of the Asu produced the first genuine military physicians and the first military medical corps for which we have evidence.

As noted earlier, the general social status of the Asu declined during the Assyrian period as a strong strain of mysticism emerged within the physician-priesthood. Less is known about the Asu's training during this period than what took place in ancient Sumer. It seems clear that copying texts remained part of the Asu's education, but one authority suggests that this activity also declined as the Asu more often transmitted their medical skills orally.[37] The existence of the term *Asu agasgu,* or "apprentice physician," suggests that the apprenticeship program was still in existence. Perhaps the medical profession as a whole was simply becoming more specialized, a development first seen under Hammurabi when he began the process of centralizing the state in 1792 BCE. If so, the Asu assumed a less prominent role in the general practice of medicine. Whatever the case, the practice of clinical medicine did not die out but continued until the end of the empire.

In Assyria, the practice of medicine was centered on the palace, and from ancient times priest-physicians attended the king, his family, and high-ranking officers and accompanied the king in the field.[38] This presence, however, would not constitute a military medical service since the physicians had no institutional support within the military bureaucracy. Moreover, this practice neither systematized the delivery of military medical care on a regular basis nor addressed the most pressing medical needs of an army, that is, the care of the troops. For a medical service to develop, it was necessary for the military to establish a mechanism for utilizing military doctors on a full-time basis. It was the low social status of the Asu, along with the organizational sophistication of the military establishment, that allowed the Assyrians to develop the first genuine military medical service.

Assyrian society was divided into three classes: the *awelu* (freemen), the *wardu* (slaves), and the *mushkenum* (plebians or commoners).[39] The last term seems to have designated some kind of military or state dependent who performed duties for the state, the most pressing of which was military service, in return for pay and certain privileges.[40] The earlier Code of Hammurabi mentions a practice called *Ilkum* in which persons of certain professions received land, grain, sheep, cattle, and other rewards from the king in return for performing services to the state or military.[41] The people named as belonging to these institutions are sailors, gendarmes, and other low-level governmental functionaries.[42] Hammurabi attempted to identify professions that were regarded as too important to allow its members to go unregulated as part of his larger plan to formalize and centralize monarchical power in Babylonia. These Ilkum were bound by an oath of obedience (the *adu*) to ensure their compliance.[43] Conscripts drawn from all classes of society also took an oath, called the *sab sharri,* that bound them to military service and the king. While it is unknown which of these oaths the Asu took, it seems likely that the Asu were regarded as an important asset to the military and formed the spine of the Assyrian military medical service. Meanwhile, the priest-physicians practiced their more magical medicine on the king and higher officers.

The Assyrian military surgeon was a product of a military state that recognized the importance of providing medical care for its soldiers. Having established and garrisoned a large number of permanent forts throughout the empire brought into being the career military physician, who was bound by oath to military service and to provide medical care to the troops. Part-time civilian physicians could no longer effectively serve the large Assyrian army, and the far-flung peacetime garrisons required the doctors to serve a tour of duty on a regular basis. There is evidence that the military doctor may have been a direct representative of the king in much the same way as the famous *musarkisus* (horse quartermasters) were.[44] The Asu were subject to the normal military chain of command and usual reporting requirements of special military personnel.

The military physician's responsibilities included caring for the wounded and maintaining the general fitness of the soldiers in garrison. Shalmaneser III's chronicle, noted earlier, suggests that these physicians also had a role in burying the dead. As in modern times, the Assyrian military doctor examined

prisoners of war. Given the labor-intensive Assyrian economy, which depended heavily on captured slave labor, this role was important. Military physicians
then attended the labor crews used in the construction and maintenance of the
irrigation system that was so vital to the Assyrians' economic survival.

The military physician also played an important medical role in the movement of foreign populations within the empire. The Assyrians routinely practiced deportation of recalcitrant peoples as a matter of state policy. Some idea
of the importance of the military physician can be gauged from the size of
these deportations. Whole towns and districts were often emptied of their
inhabitants, who were then resettled in distant regions. People who were forc-
ibly brought from other countries or other parts of the empire replaced the
deported. In 741–742 BCE, for example, 30,000 Syrians from the Hama region were sent to the Zagros Mountains, while 18,000 Aramaeans from the left
bank of the Tigris were transferred to northern Syria.[45] In 744 BCE, 65,000
people were displaced in a single operation, and the following year 154,000
people were moved from southern Mesopotamia.[46] After Sennacherib's defeat
of the Babylonians in 703 BCE, no fewer than 208,000 people were deported
from the area.[47] While the army carried out these deportations, military physicians went along to ensure that regulations governing public and military
hygiene were enforced.[48]

While no written evidence shows that the Assyrian medical corps constituted a special branch or service or that it enforced field hygiene, still, it seems
clear that the military physician must have played some role in ensuring the
provision of sanitation facilities in the field. Assyrian doctors, like their Sumerian forebears, possessed a good clinical understanding of the connection
between certain conditions and disease. The injunctions to guard against flies
and mosquitoes as causes of illness and disease are old and appear often in Sumerian and Babylonian medical literature.[49] Moreover, Assyrian doctors were
familiar with the notion that disease could spread from one person to another.
Finally, the use of lavatories was widespread in Assyria. They have been found
in the king's palace and routinely in middle-class homes.[50] That they should
not have been present in permanent military garrisons would have been un-
usual. While there is no evidence of a military sanitary corps per se, as found in
Hebraic medical literature, it is highly probable that the Asu were responsible
for ensuring the troops' military hygiene while in garrison and on campaign.

The Assyrian experience with epidemics among troop and civilian populations is well documented in numerous court records of the empire.[51] The Assyrians also dealt with epidemics on campaign and during siege operations. One example is taken from Sennacherib's campaign in Egypt. Encamped thirty miles east of Suez and awaiting further movement against the Egyptian army, Sennacherib's troops were struck by a ravaging disease. The incident must have been devastating indeed, for it is recorded in three separate sources. According to the Bible, Sennacherib's forces were ravaged "by the angel of the Lord, who went out at night and smote one hundred four score and five thousand." Herodotus says that the disease was caused by "a legion of rats gnawing everything in the weapons that was made of rope or leather," and the priest Berossus indicates that the disease was "a pestilential sickness." Whatever the cause, the effect was disastrous, and the disease killed "185,000 men with their commanders and officers."[52]

Another aspect of military medicine important to ancient armies was the veterinary doctor. The economies and military establishments of the ancient world relied heavily on animals. The Assyrians were the first to deploy large cavalry forces, and their logistics system used donkeys, horses, mules, and camels. These circumstances made proper animal care even more important. Although there is no evidence from which to discern the Assyrian veterinarian's training, it was likely the same as the Asu's with some sort of specialization in animal science. Record of the veterinary doctor appeared first in early Sumer, and the Hammurabic Code governing medical practice lists two entries regulating the behavior of veterinarians.[53] A letter from the Assyrian king Esarhaddon (680–669 BCE) mentions veterinarians among craftsmen and specialists deported from Egypt to Assyria.[54] Modern scholarship has revealed that a number of medicines and compounds that the Asu used were also prescribed and administered to animals.[55]

The appearance of the full-time military doctor integrated into the Assyrian army's overall organization is regarded as one of the more important innovations in military history. This development owes more to the level of organizational sophistication evident in all areas of Assyrian life than it does to any increase in medical knowledge. The Assyrians did not bequeath any important new medical knowledge or any new treatments to future civilizations that would have been effective in dealing with battle wounds. For the most part, Assyrian medicine was largely as effective (or ineffective) as it had been for the previous two thousand years. Nonetheless, the Assyrians were the first army in the ancient world to establish a full-time professional military medical corps and to extend routine medical treatment to their soldiers.

Unfortunately, the Assyrian innovations in military medical care died with the empire when a coalition of military forces extinguished it in 612 BCE.[56] The armies that followed Assyria, as well as most of the societies that gave them life, were not as well organized or so thoroughly integrated as the Assyrian army had been. Deprived of organizational support, the embryonic profession of the military surgeon disappeared and did not reemerge until Roman times when the imperial legions, themselves supremely organized for war, reinvented it. The armies of Persia and Greece had military surgeons attending them, but neither civilization established a professional medical service or displayed a level of organizational coherence necessary to establish and maintain a medical corps.

The medical tradition of Sumer-Babylon-Assyria that extended for more than two millennia died with the destruction of the Assyrian state. The great library of Ashurbanipal, its thousands of medical texts destroyed by fire in 612 BCE, was left to ruin, and its contents were not rediscovered until the mid-nineteenth century.[57] Because of their legendary cruelty, perhaps no people were hated more in the ancient world than the Assyrians. Retaliation was brutal, swift, and total when Assyria finally met its end. Almost all vestiges of its culture and social institutions were destroyed forever. A once clearly defined culture almost disappeared from the face of the earth. The cuneiform method of writing on clay tablets gave way to Aramaic written on papyrus, and the new language and writing methods did much to reduce the transmissibility of the long tradition of empirical medicine that Assyria had inherited. The absorption of what was once Assyria into the Persian Empire presented what was left of Assyria with a cultural challenge that it could not withstand. All these factors contributed to the dissolution of both the clinical tradition of Assyrian medicine and the innovative institution of a professional military medical corps, now dead appendages on the corpse of a nation that had once been the envy of the civilized world.

Notes

1. Roux, *Ancient Iraq*, 223–32.
2. Ibid., 228.
3. Ibid., 256.
4. A. Leo Oppenheim, *Ancient Mesopotamia: Portrait of a Dead Civilization* (Chicago: University of Chicago Press, 1977), 296.
5. A. Leo Oppenheim, "Mesopotamian Medicine," *Bulletin of the History of Medicine* 35, no. 2 (March–April 1962): 100. See also Roux, *Ancient Iraq*, 231–32.
6. Oppenheim, *Ancient Mesopotamia*, 299.
7. Garrison, *Introduction to the History of Medicine*, 62.
8. McGrew, *Encyclopedia of Medicine*, 186. See also Levey, "Some Objective Factors of Babylonian Medicine," 61–64.
9. Majno, *Healing Hand*, 40. Basic sources on Assyrian medicine include Georges Contenau, *La Médicine en Assyria et en Bablonie* (Paris: Librairie Maloine, 1938); R. Campbell Thompson, *Assyrian Medical Texts* (London: John Bale and Sons, 1924); D. D. Luckenbill, "Assyrian Drugs and Medicine," *American Journal of Semitic Languages and Literatures* 42, no. 2 (January 1926): 138–39; and Barbara Bock, "On Medicine and Magic in Ancient Mesopotamia," *Journal of Near Eastern Studies* 62, no. 1 (January 2003): 1–16.
10. Ibid.
11. Ibid.
12. Garrison, *Introduction to the History of Medicine*, 63.
13. Levey, "Some Objective Factors of Babylonian Medicine," 65.
14. Ibid., 67.
15. A. Leo Oppenheim, "Medicine in Babylonia and Assyria," in *Ancient Mesopotamia*, 101. See also, Roux, *Ancient Iraq*, 215. The most recent work on the subject of Assyrian and Babylonian medicine is Jo Anne Scurlock and Burton R. Andersen, trans., *Diagnoses in Assyrian and Babylonian Medicine: Ancient Sources, Translations, and Modern Medical Analyses* (Urbana: University of Illinois Press, 2005).
16. Levey, "Some Objective Factors of Babylonian Medicine," 67.
17. Ibid., 68.
18. Oppenheim, "Mesopotamian Medicine," 103.
19. Biggs, "Medicine in Ancient Mesopotamia," 101.
20. Garrison, *Introduction to the History of Medicine*, 63.
21. Biggs, "Medicine in Ancient Mesopotamia," 101.
22. Oppenheim, "Mesopotamian Medicine," 103.
23. Ibid., 100. See also Majno, *Healing Hand*, 48.
24. Examples of Assyrian medical primitiveness are evident in R. Campbell Thompson, "Assyrian Prescriptions for Treating Bruises and Swellings," *American Jour-*

nal of Semitic Languages and Literatures 47, no. 1 (October 1930): 1–25; by the same author, "Assyrian Prescriptions for Diseases of the Head," *American Journal of Semitic Languages and Literatures* 24, no. 1 (October 1907): 323–53; and W. G. Lambert, "A Middle Assyrian Medical Text," *Iraq* 31, no. 1 (Spring 1969): 28–39.

25. Olmstead, *History of Assyria*, 64.
26. Saggs, "Assyrian Warfare in the Sargonid Period," 145.
27. Roux, *Ancient Iraq*, 274.
28. Olmstead, *History of Assyria,* 607–8.
29. Gabriel, *Culture of War*, 60.
30. Ferrill, *Origins of War*, 145.
31. Dupuy, *Evolution of Weapons and Warfare*, 10.
32. Roux, *Ancient Iraq*, 275.
33. Ibid., 321.
34. Richard A. Gabriel, *The Great Armies of Antiquity* (Westport, CT: Praeger, 2002), 130–32; and J. N. Postgate, "The Assyrian Army at Zamua," *Iraq* 62 (2000): 89–108.
35. Ibid.
36. Laffont, *Ancient Art of Warfare*, 45.
37. Oppenheim, "Mesopotamian Medicine," 104.
38. Oppenheim, *Ancient Mesopotamia*, 304.
39. Roux, *Ancient Iraq*, 191.
40. Ibid., 193.
41. Ibid.
42. Ibid.
43. Ibid., 318.
44. See Ferrill, *Origins of War*, 72, for the role of the king's special representatives in the Assyrian state and army.
45. Roux, *Ancient Iraq*, 284.
46. Ibid.
47. Ibid., 296.
48. Adamson, "The Military Surgeon," 44. See also H. W. F. Saggs, "The Nimrud Letters," *Iraq* 36, part 9 (1974): 199–212.
49. Garrison, *Notes on the History of Military Medicine*, 28.
50. Roux, *Ancient Iraq*, 202–5.
51. Biggs, "Medicine in Ancient Mesopotamia," 97.
52. Roux, *Ancient Iraq*, 295–96.
53. Majno, *Healing Hand*, 46.
54. Biggs, "Medicine in Ancient Mesopotamia," 98.
55. Ibid.

56. Adamson, "The Military Surgeon," 44–45.
57. Ashurbanipal's library was rediscovered in 1849 by Sir Henry Layard. The first attempts to translate the documents therein appeared in print in 1914, and the task of translating the medical texts continues to this day. The collection of tablets is housed in the British Museum.

6

Israel and Persia, 1300–100 BCE

The culture of the ancient Israelites has had an enormous impact on the culture of the West. The Israelites occupy an important place in time and geography in the larger military medical developments that occurred in the Middle East between the sixth century BCE and the ascendancy of Greece and Rome. The interaction between Israelite medical practitioners and Hellenic medicine, and their experience in the Persian Empire, formed one of the main transmission belts of medical knowledge to the West. Moreover, the ability of the Hebrews to write left a relatively clear record of the role of general medicine and military medicine as they developed in the Hebraic culture of the time.

The earliest roots of Hebraic medicine are found in the biblical saga of the Israelites and their exodus from Egypt under the direction of Moses sometime in the late thirteenth century BCE. Moses was motivated by a desire to construct a new type of social order, one in which all men were priests and each had a direct relationship with a monotheistic god. The laws of the state as well as those governing social intercourse in everyday life were believed to emanate directly from the word of God. The Israelites' idea of a chosen people, hardly unique to the ancient Hebrews, implied the ability to construct a social order as a direct response to the spoken word of the deity.[1] Thus, the utterances of the deity became not only the supreme divine law but also the civic law by which the state was organized and operated in the secular sphere.

The primary influence that shaped the development of Hebraic medicine in the ancient period was the assertion of the deity as recorded in Exodus 15:26 that "I am the Lord your physician."[2] In Deuteronomy 32:39 the deity asserts further, "I wound and I heal; and there is none that can deliver you out of my hand." In this early Hebraic view, physicians were unnecessary since they could do nothing to prevent or cure disease, illness, and death, which God visited upon humans because of their sinfulness, breaking of taboo, or failure to observe ritual.[3] This medical fatalism was common among all peoples of the Middle East. But by 1500 BCE in Sumer, Babylon, and Egypt, it had been modified to allow for human intervention during illness. The basic assumption of ancient societies was that man could prevent certain things from happening to him by modifying his behavior toward the gods. Once they made this philosophical leap, it was but a short step to developing a rudimentary medical empiricism that led eventually to the emergence of the independent medical traditions in Sumer, Egypt, and Assyria. In the Israelites' case, however, a tribal people considerably less developed in many aspects of social, economic, and political maturation than were other peoples of the region at this time, the idea that human action could change one's fate at the hands of the deity emerged much later.

There is little evidence of physicians in the early days of the Israelite saga. Only a few biblical passages from this formative period mention doctors, and then they do so only in passing and not positively. They refer to apothecaries and professional midwives but offer no evidence of a medical profession per se. In preparing for the Exodus, Moses appointed his brother, Aaron, to oversee the dietary and cleanliness laws that Moses had proscribed, an event sometimes taken to mean evidence of the first public health officials in the ancient world. But Aaron was a priest and not a public official, and the basic Hebraic idea of medicine remained consistent with the view that God caused or cured illness.

The role of independent medical practitioners in the earliest period of Hebraic medicine is obscure. Simon Levin suggests that the practice of medicine in this period may have been limited to doctors treating only "surgical injuries," by which he means those cases that clearly had no religious cause.[4] This view has its parallels in Assyro-Babylonian and Egyptian medicine and may well have occurred among the Israelites as well. The belief that God caused illness for moral transgressions can only be maintained for those conditions for which a direct human cause was not readily apparent. In the case of routine injuries whose cause was hardly mysterious, including battle wounds, it is probable that their treatment could have been left to nonreligious medical practitioners as they were in Egypt and Babylon. That the Bible does not record a single instance of a priest visiting a sick person to attend to an illness suggests, albeit indirectly, that the practice of clinical medicine was not part of the social role of the temple priests. In Egypt and Babylon this priestly absence led to the emergence of a tradition of clinical pragmatism. In the case of the Israelites, however, no such pragmatic tradition emerged prior to the third century BCE.

The first mention in the Old Testament of anyone visiting a physician occurs around 900 BCE, or three hundred years after the death of Moses. King Asa of Judah seems to have suffered from an arteriosclerotic disease that caused gangrene of the feet. The Bible records that for treatment, Asa "sought not the Lord . . . but the physicians," implying the presence of medical practitioners who were independent of the temple priests.[5] Two hundred years later, the Bible records other examples of someone seeking out a physician for treatment. King Joram was wounded in battle against the Syrians and traveled to the Jezreel Valley to receive the medical attention of doctors.[6] In the same century, King Hezekia is noted as having visited doctors and using medicines they supplied to heal his illness.[7]

The only other reference to medical treatment by Hebraic physicians concerns the prophet Elijah, who seems to have practiced medicine as well as prophecy.[8] The Bible records that Elijah revived a boy who had been overcome by heatstroke, made polluted water potable (perhaps by adding salt and boiling it), made poisoned food edible, transferred leprosy from one person to another, and "smote a hostile company with blindness."[9] Whatever Elijah did, it seems to have involved at least some elements of pragmatic medicine.

Evidence of Hebraic medical practices remains sparse until at least the third century BCE, and then there are only a few references to medicine. Most of what has passed for Hebraic medicine can be found in the Talmud, a collection of commentaries written much later than the Bible. An increase in medical knowledge is reflected in both the Palestinian Talmud (370–390 CE) and the Babylonian Talmud (352–427 CE), but the medical knowledge they contain is limited and confounded by religious belief. These documents were written after three significant events in Jewish history: the Babylonian captivity, the Hellenic Greeks' three-hundred-year occupation of Israel, and the

Roman occupation of Israel and widespread assimilation of the Jews into the Roman imperium.

These events brought the Jews into direct contact with more advanced medical traditions from which they could have been expected to learn. However, the Talmud still reflects primitive medical knowledge even at this late date, confirming the power of religious belief in curtailing medical knowledge among the Hebrews. It is not until 200 BCE that one finds even faint praise for Hebraic physicians in the Talmud when Ben Sira says, "Honor a physician according to thy need for him, for verily the Lord had created him."[10] At about the same time, there appears the first evidence of specialized medical training for Jewish doctors.[11]

One interesting example of the transfer of medical concepts from Babylon to Israel is evident. The Hebraic belief that God caused illness and disease had no room for demons. The Hebrew god needed no intermediaries to work his will, and only a few references to the role of demons causing disease appear in the Mosaic phase of the Old Testament.[12] Once the Hebrews were exposed to the medical thinking in Babylon and Assyria, however, references to demons as causes of disease increase markedly in Hebraic literature.[13] This development is hardly surprising in light of the Assyro-Babylonian fixation with demons as the causes of illness.[14] In the Hebrew version of this belief, only the monotheistic god sends forth demons; by contrast, the many gods of Assyria and Babylon used demons as their minions of disease. Even in the early Christian era, one still finds a strong emphasis on the role of demons in Hebraic medicine as the cause of disease. Paradoxically, this belief occurs at a time when Greece and Rome had developed an empirical medical approach and practice to which the Jews had been exposed. An emphasis on devils and demons strongly marked early Christianity and Christian medical practice until the end of the Middle Ages.[15]

Hebraic clinical medical practice never achieved the levels seen earlier in Egypt or Babylon. The only surgical procedure mentioned in the Bible is circumcision. A Sumerian from Ur, Abraham cannot be credited with introducing circumcision to the Israelites because neither the Sumerians nor the Babylonians practiced it. Circumcision is probably more a Mosaic adoption of the Egyptian practice. Moreover, the purpose of circumcision, as with so much Hebraic medicine, was not medical at all but ritual. From ancient times, the foreskins of male children were offered as sacrifice instead of animals, a practice that testifies to its primary ritualistic rather than medical value in the Israelite tradition. The Israelites regarded circumcision as the sign of being a special class of people chosen by God. In Egypt, circumcision was generally limited to the pharaohs and nobles of the realm, a special class of men who carried the physical mark as a sign of their status. Under Joshua, however, circumcision acquired a distinct military identification when he ordered the entire Israelite male population of military age circumcised at Shittim prior to crossing the River Jordan and beginning his campaign to conquer Canaan. From then forward, circumcision was regarded in the Hebraic tradition as a sign of the covenant between the Israelites and Yahweh Saboath, their warrior god.[16]

Some idea of the Hebraic surgical skill is noted in the ritual. While Egyptian surgeons carried out circumcision with bronze or iron knives, the Hebrews continued to use a flint knife until well into Talmudic days. The usual Egyptian practice was to remove sufficient skin from the penis to expose the glans. The Egyptians had perfected the use of cautery and the hot knife during surgery and would not have found bleeding and infection a significant problem during the process. Lacking these instruments and procedures, Hebrew priests, meanwhile, removed a much smaller section of skin. This procedure made medical sense since the difficulties of controlling associated bleeding and infection were not as acute.

The only other medical implement mentioned in the Bible, the roller bandage, was used to treat a fracture of the arm. The Israelites were surely aware of this Egyptian innovation.

Hebraic medical tradition is also noteworthy for its lack of a significant materia medica. As long as two millennia before the settlement of the Israelites in Canaan, the Sumerians had developed an extensive list of drugs, poultices, and other botanical and chemical compounds used to deal with illness and injury. Certainly the Assyro-Babylonian and Egyptian drug lists were equally extensive. The failure of the Jews to develop an adequate materia medica suggests once again a powerful priesthood hindered the development of an independent branch of pragmatic medicine. The few compounds mentioned in the Bible as having medical use are olive oil, pomegranates, wormwood, cassia, poppy, mandrake, cumin for curry, myrrh, balm, and frankincense. Only myrrh is attributed with a medical use. It had such diverse applications as salve for ulcers, eye ointment, mouthwash, and enemas.[17] Unlike the practice in Babylon, Jewish practitioners refused to include animal and human dung in their medicants. The idea, Babylonian in origin, was apparently to insult the demon so that it would leave and take the disease with it.[18]

Among the more critical aspects of Hebraic medicine was the failure to develop the concept of infection. The commentators of the Bible were aware that wounds could become horribly infected ("his wound stinketh"), but they never saw this process as anything that could be prevented or dealt with by clinical means. Unlike earlier medical cultures that recognized infection as a condition that could be prevented or remedied, Hebraic medicine saw infection as a curse sent by God. The inability to deal with infection probably meant that Israelite armies suffered more deaths from infected battle wounds than the armies of Egypt or Assyria did.

The dominant role that priests played in Israelite and later Jewish society clearly had the effect of limiting the secular physician's function and greatly hindered the advancement of clinical medical knowledge and practice. Two paradoxes resulted from this state of affairs. First, priests who enforced the dietary and hygienic codes of Hebraic society also had the responsibility for ensuring a healthy public food supply. As the laws for ensuring the sanitation of the food supply were the same as for ensuring that animals used for religious sacrifice were healthy, Hebraic priests became expert in the anatomy and pathology of animals and produced an extensive literature on the subject. Unfortunately, there is no evidence that this knowledge of animal disease and pathology was extrapolated to include investigations into medical conditions afflicting the human body or that the priests shared their knowledge with practicing physicians.

A second paradox resulting from the dominance of the priestly caste was that the only physicians in full-time practice and paid by the state were the doctors providing medical care to the priests. The primacy of religion precluded the development of an independent medical profession to serve the general populace even though this same primacy brought full-time medical practitioners into service to the priests. The priests' responsibility to determine the purity of animals for sacrifice, meanwhile, turned the temples into virtual slaughterhouses. The constant need to dissect and examine the internal organs of these animals put the priests at great and continuous risk of enteritis and other diseases.[19] To deal with this medical risk, the priests followed the same route as King Asa, who "sought not the Lord . . . but physicians." Thus the priests who lectured the populace to rely on priests to cure disease and illness employed full-time physicians to deal with their own ills.

All aspects of Hebraic medical knowledge and practice from the time of Moses to at least the second century BCE were generally far less than those found in the other states of the area during the same period. Hebraic surgery was primitive by Egyptian standards, as was the skill to treat routine injuries. As noted, the only effective empirical medical device recorded in the Bible, the roller bandage, is clearly an Egyptian contribution. Hebraic knowledge of drugs and other medicinals was also extremely limited, and its materia medica was far less comprehensive than that of Sumer or Babylon. For all practical purposes, then, the ancient Hebrews never developed a clinical theory of illness and disease and instead relied entirely on religious explanations and cures. After the Babylonian captivity, Hebrew theories of disease included the demons for which Babylonian medicine was famous but to no pragmatic effect. Hebraic medicine never developed the idea, central to any medical progress, that man could control his own medical fate through empirical observation and practice. Jewish doctors received no medical training until well into the Alexandrian period, and the profession of medicine never established a truly independent and important role for itself. As a consequence, Hebraic medicine contributed virtually nothing to the medical knowledge of the ancient world.

The Hebraic contribution to medical knowledge as a whole may have been minimal, but its contribution to military medicine was significant. In the early Israelite armies, the world finds the first organized military medical sanitary corps in ancient times. Although they were priests and not military physicians, these medical officers came under military command during times of war. Further, although the impulse was religious and not medical, the temple priests' enforcement of strict hygiene standards in the military constituted a significant military asset for Israelite armies. In this regard, it is wise to recall that even today the military doctor's role is not so much humanitarian as it is pragmatic; that is, the doctor ensures that as many personnel as possible are retained as combat assets by reducing disease and repairing the wounded.

An interesting aspect of the early Israelite military sanitary corps is that it emerged within a military organization that was far less developed than those found in Sumer, Egypt, Babylon, and Assyria. The highest period of military organizational development of Hebraic armies was reached under King David (1005–961 BCE) and King Solomon (961–921 BCE). The Davidic armies were militia armies trained and commanded by a small, regular force that served as permanent cadre to lead the conscripts when called to service. This cadre was made up of the *gibborim* (mighty men), who were proven combat warriors, and a corps of mercenary troops, most notably Philistines, who were equipped with heavier armament than were the Israelites.[20] The conscript force was called for military service in tribal segments, with each segment serving one month of active duty at a time; however, in wartime the entire national force might be called to arms. This rotation of reserve forces is still seen today in the Israeli Defense Force and for the same reason: prolonged periods of military duty for large segments of the population would have meant severe economic disruption, especially in an agricultural economy.

The Israelite army was essentially an infantry force, a fact noted in the biblical accounts of warfare where men are ordered to "run before the king." Armed with spears and swords made of bronze, the centerpiece of these armies was the heavy infantry. There is, however, some evidence that a mix of lighter forces—archers, slingers, and javelin throwers—augmented the heavy infantry.[21] Under Solomon, Israelite armies acquired a chariot corps largely of experienced Philistine charioteers and machines. Chariot units were stationed at key points throughout the country in what the Bible calls chariot cities.[22] Israelite tactical organization seems to have persisted along early Mosaic lines. Units were divided into hundreds, fifties, and tens, and each had its own "captain." A number of battle accounts record that units were formed into battalions of six hundred men, perhaps suggesting that these battalions were the basic combat units of the army.[23] The size of these Davidic and Solomonic armies is not revealed in the biblical accounts, but it is hardly likely that even at maximum mobilization these armies could have sustained a force of more than ten thousand to fifteen thousand men in the field for very long.[24]

The origins of the military sanitation corps are found in the Exodus saga. Moses set strict dietary and hygienic laws whose observance came to define membership in the Jewish people.[25] The value of these dietary and hygienic laws lay principally in their cultic role in defining the Israelites as a separate people. Only secondarily do the dietary laws have any medical value.[26] The hygienic laws, of course, although promulgated for religious reasons, do have great medical value. A number of these hygienic laws were also designed to regulate social behavior, especially sexual behavior. Many of them—especially the proscriptions against abortion, coitus interruptus, bestiality, homosexuality, and so on—were passed to the West, where they later became the basis for the first medical jurisprudence.[27]

The hygienic laws constituted a form of preventive medicine. Like any good physician, Moses recognized that it is far easier to prevent an epidemic than to stop one once it is under way. The complete list of dietary and hygienic laws is found in Leviticus, which may have been written much later but redacted to imply a Mosaic origin. An informative passage in Deuteronomy 23:9–14 lays out the rules for keeping a military camp clean: "If there be any among you any man, that is not clean by reason of uncleanness that chanceth him by night, then shall go abroad out of the camp, he shall not come within the camp again." The injunction mandates that if a man falls ill, he is to be housed outside the camp until the illness passes. The afflicted soldier is to remain outside the camp for seven days, and the priest must go outside the camp to inspect the soldier. Even on the march, the sick soldier had to remain behind the column, keeping up as best he could. These practices were an effective way of preventing contagion, and the Bible mentions they were to be enforced whenever leprosy, rash, or discharge [infection?] was evident.[28] Elsewhere, it was prescribed that persons or families struck by disease were to be quarantined for as long as forty days.[29] If the disease did not abate, the houses, clothes, and possessions of the sick were to be "purified" first by washing and, if need be, by destroying the house with fire. In some instances the walls of the house were to be scrubbed clean with "fair water," a reference to boiling water. These same procedures were used in military camps.

The Bible dictated additional hygiene practices that were related to military life. Deuteronomy 23:13–14 required sanitary habits that often were not practiced by European armies until World War I: "Further, there shall be an area for you outside the camp, where you may relieve yourself." Separating the latrine from the camp and, most important, from the water supply was frequently not done even during the American Civil War. But alone, separation was not sufficient. Deuteronomy goes on to say, "With your gear you shall have a spike [probably a small shovel], and when you have squatted you shall dig a hole with it to cover up your excrement." These two practices must have done much to reduce the rate and spread of disease in Israelite armies. The Israelites recognized that disease could also be spread through contaminated objects such as clothing, blankets, woven material, and saddles. These items had to be washed before the recovered soldiers were allowed to return to camp. The injunctions to wash one's hands before eating or after toileting and to wash one's body and clothes frequently were also excellent military hygiene practices, but they would have been of only limited value without a genuine disinfectant soap.

Numbers 31:19–24 outlines procedures for dealing with battle casualties. Anyone who killed a man in battle or touched a corpse had to remain outside the camp for seven days. While the origin of the corpse taboo was religious,[30] its practical effect was to reduce contagion by quarantining soldiers who had been exposed to blood, a common disease source. Ancient battles often involved close combat during which blood might have easily splattered on the soldier.[31] This concern is also reflected in the need to purify any weapons and clothing that have been exposed to blood. Metal weapons—"whatever can stand fire"—were required to be purified by fire. Other equipment, including booty, had to be washed before it could be brought into the camp.

Strict rules dictated how to handle the dead, and the law provided for a quick burial. The ancient Israelites apparently buried their dead outside the city walls or the military camp. Israelite hygienic practices also required that no well be dug near a cemetery. Water had to be boiled prior to drinking whenever there was any doubt of its cleanliness, and water left uncovered was considered unfit to consume.[32] Given the number of waterborne diseases that crippled or destroyed armies over the centuries, ensuring the cleanliness of the water supply as a regular military habit was a major military innovation.

The prescription of dietary laws and hygienic practices would have been a major military asset provided they were consistently followed. Placing the enforcement of these regulations in the hands of priests who accompanied the army probably ensured that the rules were sufficiently enforced. Even so, like all ancient peoples, the ancient Israelites lived in fear of epidemic, and during the Exodus under the careful eyes of Moses and his chief health officer, Aaron, the tribe still suffered several epidemics. Particularly feared it seems was diphtheria (*eschara*). The law required that after three cases of infectious disease were reported in the community, the *shofar*, or "warning horn," had to be blown to alert people of an epidemic. So feared was diphtheria, however, that the law prescribed that the shofar be sounded at the discovery of the first case of the disease.[33] The degree of success in preventing disease by these dietary and hygienic regulations cannot be estimated. It is certainly possible that they had a generally beneficial effect, but at least one authority suggests that the practical difficulties in observing these laws on a daily basis, as well as the low quality of general health in the ancient world, probably made them less effective than they would have been in later times.[34]

Nonetheless, the creation of a military sanitary corps was a genuine innovation that can be attributed to the armies of ancient Israel. The goal was no less than ensuring pure food, clean water, a disease-free military camp, and general good health for the soldier to enable him to remain an effective combat asset. The hygienic corps of the Israelites can be seen as the formalization and institutionalization of similar cultic practices evident in Babylon and Egypt. But it is precisely the formalization and institutionalization within the army that made them innovative. This said, the idea of a military sanitary corps was hardly an immediate success. The Persian armies practiced a form of ritual hygiene similar to that of the Jews but lacked the strong degree of religious enforcement necessary to make it work effectively. The armies of classical Greece had no sanitary corps or field hygiene regulations at all, and there is no evidence of these regulations in Alexandrian armies. The armies of Rome, however, raised military hygiene to heights far beyond those of any ancient army, but the practice died with the collapse of the empire. The numerous accounts of armies ravaged by easily preventable diseases up through the Middle Ages seem sufficient proof of the valuable contribution the Hebraic armies made to military medicine, even if it was largely ignored by later armies.

One aspect of Hebraic military medical practice was unique. In World War II, Allied armies about to be sent into combat repeatedly screened the troops to remove potential psychiatric casualties from the ranks.[35] Israelite military commanders seem to have done the same thing in ancient times. Deuteronomy 20:5–9 instructs troop commanders to take out certain kinds of people from the fighting ranks precisely because they were not likely to fight well:

The officials shall address the troops as follows: "Is there anyone who has built a new house but has not dedicated it? Let him go back to his home, lest he die in battle and another dedicate it. Is there anyone who has planted a vineyard but has never harvested it? Let him go back to his home, lest he die in battle and another harvest it. Is there anyone who has paid the bride-price for a wife, but who has not yet married her? Let him go back to his home, lest he die in battle and another marry her." The officials shall go on addressing the troops and say, "Is there anyone afraid and disheartened? Let him go back to his home, lest the courage of his comrades flag like his." When the officials have finished addressing the troops, army commanders shall assume command of the troops.

These conditions were more likely to affect young conscripts than they would the army's seasoned soldiers, who were professional warriors. The army of Israel was becoming a national army and had to deal with the problems of confidence, fighting spirit, and psychiatric collapse that had afflicted all armies from time immemorial. In requiring the priests to examine the troops according to a list of conditions that could reduce troop morale and fighting spirit, the Israelites introduced the first practical method of military psychiatric screening.[36]

Persia, 553–331 BCE

Cyrus the Great (546–528 BCE) forged the great Persian Empire, but it lasted only two centuries until the armies of Alexander the Great destroyed it at the battles of the Granicus River (334 BCE), Issus (333 BCE), and Arbela (331 BCE). Once the greatest military power of its day, its remnants were forced to endure successive foreign regimes for the next thousand years. The Macedonian Seleucid and the Parthian (Arsacid) dominations lasted for almost five hundred years (330 BCE–226 CE); were followed by the Sassanid, or neo-Assyrian, Empire (226–651 CE); and finally came under Muslim Arab control after the battle of Nehavend (641 CE). In all this time, and especially during the old empire, Persian medicine, social life, and technology lagged far behind developments in other states of the region.

Persian social structure, religion, and medicine remained closely intertwined from the beginning, acting as reciprocal forces in the development of Persian culture. The empire's essentially tribal and nomadic social organization strongly reinforced the traditional religious beliefs that dominated the country during its tribal period, and, in turn, religion strongly influenced the development of medicine. As a consequence, "through the whole history of the Persian people up to the Arabic period, never a trace of rational treatment or prevention of disease by simple natural means is discernible."[37] The only available sources from which to discern Persian medical practice are religious books.[38]

Religion and medicine in Persia had their roots in the original Aryan migration from Central Asia, when Hindu and Persian strains formed a common population stock. Around 1600 BCE the Indian Aryans occupied the Punjab in one of the many migratory movements of the day. Some of the region's resident tribes were forced south into the land area now known as Persia. These people called themselves Airya, and the name of the high plateau where they settled became known as Ayrana or Iran, the home of the Aryans. The people who eventually came to be called Persians were only one of the many Aryan tribes of the area. Others, such as the Medes, Parthians, and Bactrians, were eventually subsumed under Persian rule, but they never lost their cultural identity and reappeared from time to time as distinct entities in the country. Persia always was and largely remained a multitribal state, a fact that shaped the empire's political and military structures and institutions and imposed severe limits on developments in other areas, including medicine.

These centripetal and centrifugal forces within Persian culture and society were in constant tension throughout the imperial period. In 546 BCE Cyrus II, or Cyrus the Great, acceded to the Persian throne. In a series of wars, he conquered the Medes in 549 BCE to form the first Persian Empire. As only one tribe in a larger coalition of tribes, even the Persians were governed by an alliance of seven royal families of which the Achaemenians were the first among equals. Tribal wars occupied far more of the emperor's time than foreign conquests, and Persian political and military policy alternated between wars against foreigners and wars against internal tribes in open rebellion.

In 522 BCE Darius I, or Darius the Great, faced the problem of governing an empire that comprised no fewer than forty-seven different tribal nations.[39] To enforce Persian rule, Darius established the satrap system of imperial administration that was designed to prevent the revolt of parochialism by tying the provinces tightly to the Persian center. Darius began the famous system of royal roads so that Persian troops could move quickly to quell revolts, stationed Persian national forces in the provinces, and sent Persian officers to provincial tribal armies to control training and logistics. Darius also authorized special police and intelligence units known as "eyes of the king" to watch over developments in the provinces and punish recalcitrant local officials. Even with these administrative institutions in place, however, provincial revolts were frequent. In the end, it was more the deteriorating political situation within the empire than Greek military pressure that brought down the empire.

The decentralized tribal nature of the Persian state was reflected in its military organization. Although all Persians were subject to national conscription and formed the core of the national army, the bulk of the Persian army comprised relatively independent tribal armies called to the colors in wartime. While the Persian contingents were extremely well organized, trained, and disciplined, the levied tribal forces that augmented the national army, for the most part, received only limited training, wore dissimilar uniforms or national dress, carried diverse weapons, spoke various languages, and fought in different ways. Most often these forces were commanded by their own chiefs and were not regarded as either politically or militarily reliable. It was the Persian practice to occupy the center of the line and to use Persian cavalry units in the rear and on the flanks to ensure that the tribal units did not break and run in battle.

The Persians' central hold on the centrifugal forces pulling away from the empire was always tenuous, especially with regard to medical theory and practice and the influence of tribal religions. Persian religious beliefs and rituals had their roots in the long-distant Aryan past that the Persians shared with the Indians. Both peoples had a common mythology built on fire worship and featured a sacrificial flame tended by a sacred priesthood that served multiple gods. By 1000 BCE, this common religious system broke apart, with the Persians going their own way and recasting the old gods of the Indians as demons in Persian religious thought. The Persians' religious ideas and practices remained "the rituals of a nomadic people with no local habitation, no agriculture, no stalls or stables, but forever on the move, herding cattle across the steppe" long after they had settled on the Iranian plateau.[40] The pastoral roots of Persian religion are evident in the belief that the dog, cow, and human occupied equal moral status.

Sometime in the sixth century BCE, a reformer called Zoroaster formalized the traditional religious creed and developed it around the tension between the dual forces of good and evil. By the fifth century BCE, the emperor had adopted the new religious ideas, and the Zoroastrian faith gradually spread from the court to the rest of the population. The tenets of the new creed were written in the Avesta, a collection of works similar to the Old Testament that served the same function for the Persians as the Bible did for the Hebrews.[41] Another book, the Videvdad, dealt with the law and political organization and is noteworthy for its information on hygienic laws and the role of physicians. These two books, coupled with archaeological findings and the writings of Greek commentators, constitute most of our knowledge of Persian medicine.[42]

Similar to the practices and beliefs of the ancient Hebrews, the Persians' were primarily designed to achieve religious and ritual purposes rather than medical ones, for the Persians believed in the fatality of the will of the gods against which man was powerless. Thus, while the Avesta contains admonitions to prevent disease through complex purification rituals and the use of physicians, few of these strictures are medicinal in nature.[43] And as with similar strictures found in Leviticus, their observance is left to priests and not physicians.

The powerful priesthood's strong and continued control of both the theory and practice of medicine was thoroughly integrated into every aspect of Persian life and retarded the development of any independent Persian clinical medical tradition. Not a single medical practice in ancient Persia attained a level of development above primitive folk medicine, and one searches in vain for the contributions of empirical physicians similar to those found in Sumer, Egypt, and Assyria.

Priest-physicians were trained in the temples, and the tripartite division of medical practice found in Babylon and Assyria was also evident in Persia. The Avesta describes three types of doctors: those who heal with the knife, those who heal with sacred herbs, and those who heal with the holy word. The level of surgery seems to have been confined to simple lancing of boils and abscesses, and the Persian materia medica remained decidedly primitive.[44] The *Denkart,* which is part of the Avesta, contains the assertion that Ahuramazda, the divine creative power in the universe, created ten thousand herbs for healing illness.[45] It also mentions drugs that were believed to have an anesthetic effect, including wine, opium, mandragora, poppy, hemlock, and nightshade.[46]

Yet no evidence suggests that the *Athravans* (herb doctors) ever developed a written materia medica anywhere near as extensive as those found in Egypt, Sumer, or Babylon.

Some of the temples served as medical schools for training physicians, but much of their training was centered on religious beliefs and rituals, a practice that prevented the development of an independent clinical medical tradition separate from the priesthood. Apart from the facts that surgical training required a period of apprenticeship, that surgeons were licensed, and that they could charge fees on the same basis as found in the Hammurabi Code, we have no information about the training of Persian physicians. We do know, however, that the physicians who healed with the holy word, or the priests, were the most highly regarded. Darius himself, though, seems to have relied upon more "pragmatic" physicians and employed Democedes of Samos, regarded as the greatest physician of the day, as his personal physician.

The Avesta notes the following clinical conditions but not how they were treated: blindness, deafness, lameness, epilepsy, scabies, fevers, insanity, leprosy, poisoning, snakebite, headache, various physical deformities, and toothache.[47] Therapy seems to have included mostly incantations, amulets, and various potions made from medicinal herbs. Surgery was generally confined to lancing and other minor scarifications.

Persian Military Medicine

For all the hindrances to the development of high levels of military, social, and medical organization, the Persians were first and foremost a warrior people who took great pride in their war-fighting skills. Their almost constant state of war against foreign enemies or tribal revolts must have heightened the need to develop a tradition of pragmatic medicine to serve the army. The decentralization evident in retaining forty-seven different tribal armies strongly militated against providing centralized military medical facilities. Nevertheless, the strong sense of national identity and the pride of the Persian regular national force must have prodded the king and the officer corps to some consideration of military medical care.

It is known that Darius thought highly of Egyptian physicians and regularly had them in attendance at his court. He restored the medical school at Sais for them to practice.[48] Later, when contacts with the Greeks became more extensive, Greek doctors were present at the Persian court and became serious competitors as medical practitioners. While Greek doctors could have provided the Persians with a number of empirical skills useful to the army, not having a military medical corps in the armies of classical Greece probably hindered the development of any military medical care beyond the treatment of the king and his generals. While there is evidence that the priests and physicians attended the army in battle, no evidence suggests that they were present outside the top command structure.

Meanwhile, the need to treat battle casualties remained. The Persians' experience with the armies of Egypt and Assyria, both of which had strong empirical traditions in the medical service of their military forces, would probably have picked up some of this knowledge. One authority suggests, although without hard evidence, that as great cultural borrowers the Persians would have readily incorporated into their medical establishment the extant Egyptian and Greek knowledge of how to treat battle wounds, and this information would not necessarily be reflected in the religious texts from which we obtain our knowledge of Persian medicine. The Greek commentators of the day were silent on the subject of Persian military medicine.[49]

What remains, then, is the possibility that the Persians may have borrowed some elements of the Egyptian, Assyrian, and Greek empirical tradition and perhaps employed them in some manner in the army. No evidence of any formal Persian medical service is available. Perhaps within the Persian army itself, as in the armies of Greece and the Roman Republic, soldiers gained practical medical knowledge of how to treat battle injuries and provided medical treatment on an ad hoc basis to their comrades, but no credible evidence supports these propositions.

Notes

1. The ancient idea that the commands of a deity ought to serve as the basis for civic law remains very much with us. It was the basis of the Pilgrim community in Massachusetts, John Calvin's community, and modern-day conservative Islam. Some Orthodox Jewish communities regard the state of Israel as illegitimate precisely on the grounds that it is governed by secular, not divine, law.
2. Simon S. Levin, *Adam's Rib: Essays on Biblical Medicine* (Los Altos, CA: Geron-X Press, 1970), 40.

3. Some Orthodox Jews maintain that the Holocaust was divine retribution for the change in Jewish ritual brought about by the Jewish Reform Movement.

4. Levin, *Adam's Rib*, 41. See also Maurice Bear Gordon, *Medicine among the Ancient Hebrews* (Chicago: University of Chicago Press, 1941); his work is summarized in an article by the same title and appears in *Isis* 33, no. 4 (December 1941): 454–85.

5. 2 Chronicles 16:12. See also Andre De Vries and Abraham Weinberger, "King Asa's Presumed Gout: A 20th Century Discussion of a 9th Century B.C. Biblical Patient," *New York State Journal of Medicine*, February 1975, 452–55. It did Asa no good. He succumbed to his illness.

6. Levin, *Adam's Rib*, 46.

7. Ibid.

8. Ibid.

9. Ibid.

10. Flavius Josephus, *Jewish Antiquities*, trans. William Whiston (London: Wordsworth Editions, 2006), 4:38:1.

11. Garrison, *Introduction to the History of Medicine*, 70.

12. During an outbreak of cholera during the Exodus, Moses drove away the demon that caused the disease with a metal serpent wrapped around a stick, giving rise to charges of idolatry. The metal serpent was nevertheless placed on the altar of the temple later built by Solomon. For more on idolatry in Judaism, see Karen Randolph Joines, "The Bronze Serpent in the Israelite Cult," *Journal of Biblical Literature* 87, no. 3 (September 1968): 245–56; and T. Witton Davies, "Magic, Divination, and Demonology among the Semites," *American Journal of Semitic Languages and Literatures* 14, no. 4 (July 1898): 241–51.

13. Levin, *Adam's Rib*, 57.

14. An excellent source of information on Assyrian and Babylonian demons as the causes of disease and other catastrophes is Jeremy Black and Anthony Green, *Gods, Demons, and Symbols of Ancient Mesopotamia: An Illustrated Dictionary* (Austin: University of Texas Press, 1992).

15. One reason for this emphasis may have been Christ's association with the Essenes, a cultic sect of Judaism noted for its asceticism and belief in demons.

16. Gabriel, *The Military History of Ancient Israel*, 129–30. See also Eric Isaac, "Circumcision as Covenant Rite," *Anthropos* 59 (1965): 444. Exodus 15:3 describes Yahweh as the Divine Warrior.

17. Levin, *Adam's Rib*, 61–62, for the Hebraic materia medica and its uses.

18. McGrew, *Encyclopedia of Medical History*, 130.

19. Leonard J. Hoenig, "Ben Achira: The First Gastroenterologist in Ancient Israel," *Gastroenterology* 11, no.1 (1989): 61–63.

20. Chaim Herzog and Mordechai Gichon, *Battles of the Bible* (Jerusalem: Steimatzky Agency Ltd., 1978), 87; and Gabriel, *Military History of Ancient Israel*,

32–34.

21. Gabriel, *Military History of Ancient Israel*, 92–93, for the mix of weapons in the Israelite army; and Herzog and Gichon, *Battles of the Bible*, 88.

22. Gabriel, *Military History of Ancient Israel*, 35–37.

23. Herzog and Gichon, *Battles of the Bible*, 89.

24. Ibid., 88.

25. Or so the order of books in the Bible would imply. In fact, however, it is more likely that the Leviticus laws did not exist during Exodus times and were formulated only after the Jews returned from exile in Babylon. Then the Jerusalem priesthood promulgated the laws as a mechanism of defining "genuine" Jews—those who had been in exile—from "others," or mostly those who had remained behind and reverted to paganism. It was this definition that permitted the returning exiles to lay claim to their former lands and properties that the pagans had taken.

26. The dietary laws promulgated in Leviticus are generally of no medical value, and there is no truth to the view that they would provide for an optimal food supply for military operations in a tropical climate. That other peoples of the region ate and mixed foods forbidden by Hebraic laws with no general ill effect seems evidence enough that the dietary laws were primarily ritualistic and not hygienic. A contrary view can be found in Charles F. Pfeiffer, ed., *The Biblical World: A Dictionary of Biblical Archaeology* (Grand Rapids, MI: Baker Book House, 1966), 373.

27. Garrison, *Introduction to the History of Medicine*, 68.

28. Gabriel, *Military History of Ancient Israel*, 92.

29. Leviticus's rules governing the hygiene of the military camp are quoted at length in Garrison, *Notes on the History of Military Medicine*, 31. More detailed references to these rules are presented in Leon Goldman, "Syphilis in the Bible," *Archaeological Dermatology* 103 (May 1971): 536. An analysis of the importance of these measures to modern field medicine can be found in Edgar Erskine Hume, *The Military Sanitation of Moses in Light of Modern Knowledge* (Carlisle Barracks, PA: Medical Field Service School, 1940). Interestingly, forty days is the same period of time that people were isolated in Venice at the height of the Black Death in Europe. The Italian word for forty is *quaranta*. It is thought that the Italians chose this length of time because it is equal to the forty days that the New Testament says Christ was in the desert.

30. The religious origin of the corpse taboo in Hebraic theology is discussed in A. S. Yahuda, "The Osiris Cult and the Designation of Osiris Idols in the Bible," *Journal of Near Eastern Studies* 3, no. 3 (1944), 194–97. The taboo has its roots in the fear of the corpse of Osiris, whose body rose from the dead. Its original intent was to prohibit the worship of Osiris by the ancient Israelites, who were familiar with the cult after their long residence in Egypt. In practice, however,

the prohibition was extended to a fear of all corpses. For more on this and other elements of Hebraic theology that have Egyptian roots, see Richard A. Gabriel, *Gods of Our Fathers: The Memory of Egypt in Judaism and Christianity* (Westport, CT: Greenwood, 2002).

31. For the blood taboo of the Israelites, see Morton Smith, *Jesus the Magician: Charlatan or Son of God?* (Berkeley, CA: Seastone, 1998).

32. McGrew, *Encyclopedia of Medical History*, 130.

33. Garrison, *Introduction to the History of Medicine*, 69.

34. Edward Neufeld, "Hygiene Conditions in Ancient Israel (Iron Age)," *Journal of the History of Medicine*, October 1970, 414–37.

35. Gabriel, *No More Heroes*, 87–88.

36. For a history of psychiatric screening in war, see ibid., chapter 4.

37. Fielding H. Garrison, "Persian Medicine and Medicine in Persia: A Geomedical Survey," *Bulletin of the History of Medicine* 1, no. 4 (May 1933): 141.

38. Henry E. Sigerist, *A History of Medicine* (New York: Oxford University Press, 1951), 199.

39. Zoka, *The Imperial Iranian Army*, 10–20. See also Gabriel, *Empires at War*, vol. 1, chapter 9, for a complete analysis of the Persian army and its nationality problem; and Gabriel, *Culture of War*, 73.

40. G. Sticker, *Essays in the History of Medicine* (London: Sudhoff-Festschrift, 1924), 8–23.

41. The best general work on ancient Persian medicine is Cyril Elgood, *Medicine in Persia* (New York: AMS Press, 1978). For the history of the Avesta, see Sindokht Dehesh, "Pre-Islamic Medicine in Persia," *Middle East Journal of Anaesthesiology* 4, no. 5 (June 1975): 377–82. Also of interest is E. Herzfeld, *Zoroaster and His World* (Princeton, NJ: Princeton University Press, 1947).

42. Sigerist, *History of Medicine*, 202.

43. It is likely that while under the Persians, the Jews acquired some of the purification rituals found in Leviticus before Cyrus released the Jews from the Babylonian captivity. The ritual where persons are sprinkled with water (Leviticus 14) may have been acquired in this manner. The Persians observed the same ritual but used cow urine.

44. See David Hooper, "Some Persian Drugs," *Bulletin of Miscellaneous Information* 31, no. 6 (1931): 299–344.

45. Dehesh, "Pre-Islamic Medicine in Persia," 380.

46. Ibid., 382.

47. Garrison, *Introduction to the History of Medicine*, 144.

48. Sigerist, *History of Medicine*, 202.

49. Ibid., 206. With the exception of a few instances where it is noted that the Persian king had physicians in attendance (*Cyropaedia*, 1, 5, 15–19), there are no references to Persian military doctors.

7

INDIA,
400–100 BCE

The primitive level of Persian medical knowledge and expertise stands in stark contrast to that of another people that resided close by and whose culture flourished at approximately the same time. A strongly empirical medical tradition became deeply integrated into the military structures of societies that flourished within the culture of the Indus and Ganges River valleys of India during the fourth century BCE. Indian medicine developed an empirical tradition of pragmatic medicine that even surpassed most elements of Greek medicine extant at the same time. Had the Greek and Indian cultures come into substantial contact, there would have been much that Indian physicians could have taught the Greeks. While the empirical medical tradition of Greece ultimately collapsed in a sea of mysticism and superstition, the Indian clinical tradition continued to develop and remains the basis for much of Indian medicine practiced today.[1]

The Indian civilization is very old. As long ago as 2500 BCE, the native, dark-skinned Indian peoples had developed a thriving culture that included their own written language in the Indus River valley.[2] About 1800 BCE, this culture was disrupted by the same Aryan invasions that ultimately resulted in the Aryan settlement of Iran by the Persians and the settlement of the Mitanni in northern Iraq. Within nine hundred years, the invaders had conquered most of India, reducing the native population to serf status and preserving their own superior social position by imposing a caste system based on skin color. Over time, however, a composite culture arose in the Indus and Ganges River valleys of northern India that came to be known as Indo-Aryan. The regions' predominantly animist and pantheistic native religions were altered by the religious and social ideas of the newcomers, who brought with them (or perhaps produced after their arrival) a large body of literature called the Vedas. This literature was embodied in four sacred books written in Sanskrit that were supposedly produced by divine inspiration sometime in the ancient past. The Vedas provided detailed instructions on many subjects, including medicine as an art practiced within a strongly religious context. The word *veda* literally means "wisdom," and the Aryan word for physician, *vaidya,* means "he who knows wisdom."[3] Although Vedic thought strongly linked medical practice with religion, it reserved a special place for the physician that was much more independently defined and allowed a broader scope for empirical experimentation and practice than did any of the other medico-religious traditions of antiquity.

The culture of the Indus Valley achieved a high degree of stability and political development, only to have its achievements overshadowed when the area was incorporated into the Persian Empire. The Persians call the Indus people Hindu because they had difficulty in pronouncing the letter *I,* and the name passed to later generations of Greek writers. Later, in 326 BCE, substantial areas of the Indus Valley came under Greek domination when Alexander brought them into the Macedonian Empire. In the Ganges Valley to the east, however, the Indo-Aryan culture remained fragmented in a number of rival kingdoms (*mahajanapadas*), each ruled by a caste of warrior aristocrats who fought frequent wars with one another. The situation was similar to the conditions in ancient Sumer, where rival city-states battled one another for centuries. Warfare seems to have been the predominant occupation of the upper classes of the Ganges Valley civilization.[4]

Warfare is a powerful stimulus to medical development, especially when the most socially prominent classes of a society are directly involved in it. Frequent wars placed a premium on developing medical skills that could be placed at the service of the army and the warrior classes that fought them. Although transmitted through the ages mainly by oral tradition, the Vedas achieved written form sometime in the sixth century BCE. The sections dealing with medicine reflect a deep concern for pragmatic medicine and clinical applications, and it is not surprising that the Vedas explain how to integrate medical practice into the military organizations of the day. Whereas Persia failed to develop an empirical medical tradition or military medical service, the Indian culture of the same period developed both to a great degree.

The history of Indian medicine can be divided into two major periods. In the earlier Vedic period (1500–800 BCE), most of the medical information and practice was derived from the Vedas. The later Brahminic period includes the interval from 800 BCE to 1000 CE, after which Indian medicine fell under the influence of the Islamic conquest and Muslim physicians took over medical practice. Initiating a great religious movement of the sixth century BCE, Buddhist teachings had an important effect on Indian medicine. During this time practitioners founded hospitals, a development that Christianity did not bring to the West for many centuries. Buddha's rejection of the caste system also led to the medical treatment of all castes, regardless of their status. Buddha was himself a prince of the *Kshatriya* (warrior) class but preached the need for mercy in war, including the obligation to treat the enemy wounded.

The Vedic system of medicine was called Ayurveda, literally "knowledge of life" or "science of life."[5] Its rules and practices were contained in the fourth Veda, or *Atharva Veda,* a collection of spells, incantations, and medicants constituting the medical lore of the Atharvan priests. Ayurvedic medicine was further codified in detail in two major treatises by Charaka and Sushruta, historical personalities shrouded in myth and mysticism. Both treatises incorporated centuries of Vedic medical knowledge and practice. (Sometime around 600 CE, a third book, the *Ashtanga Sangraha* by Vagbhata, appeared.) The *Charaka Samhita* was mainly a treatise on religious medicine, but its strong empirical emphasis provided pragmatic protocols for dealing with specific illness, diseases, and injuries. The second work, the *Sushruta Samhita,* was a treatise on clinical surgery, although it too reflects a strong religious emphasis. The earliest written records of Vedic culture were inscribed on birch bark, and little remains of these earlier texts. The dates when the samhitas were finally written is unknown, varying from as early as 1000 BCE to as late as the second century CE.[6] The religious belief that all things of this world are transitory led the Indians, especially the priestly caste, to regard permanent records as a pointless exercise in human vanity. However, the ancient practice of requiring physicians to commit these texts to memory and repeat them orally allowed their contents to survive throughout the ages, so much of their substance is retrievable.

Indian medical theory and practice evolved within the context of the social order of the Indo-Aryan societies of the first millennium BCE. These societies were warrior societies in which a strict caste system was imposed. At the top of the social order were the Brahmin priests whose claim to social status rested in their being "twice-born" and in living their second lifetime on the way to nirvana. Their strong religious orientation and the belief that good works and merit were the roads to the ultimate definition of their soul and existence made them less powerful in the day-to-day activities of the state than their religious status would suggest. Below the Brahmin priests, but clearly above them in power and social status, were the Kshatriyas, or warrior nobles, who actually governed the society and conducted its many wars. A general class of *Vaishyas* (freemen) made up the remaining bulk of the population. Within each caste were hundreds of subcastes, numbering perhaps as many as four thousand.

The organization of the Indian state is contained in a book on polity called the *Arthashastra*, a Vedic version of Aristotle's *Politics*. Some idea of the social order's military nature is reflected in its art of governing, which is called *dandaniti,* or the "science of cruelty." The book details a number of cruel punishments for social transgressions and suggests that a fundamental political principle required the use of terror or force to maintain order in the state.[7] It is unclear what influence the passive ideology of Buddhism, with its emphasis on individual spirituality and the cycle of existence, had on actual governmental practices. In all probability, the Indian social order of the Brahminic period was not as harsh as it would first appear and probably no more so than the Christian followers of Augustine found the government of Rome to be.

Perhaps no society in the ancient world was more strongly influenced by religious ideas in a general sense. All aspects of Indian social life had religious elements to govern them. In principle, if not in fact, the Brahmin priests, whose position was obtained through purely religious means, ruled the social order. The nonmaterial orientation of religious belief permitted the priesthood to regard the concerns of this life as both transitory and of little value. At the same time, however, Indian society faced the practical challenge of survival amid constant warfare, a fact that placed effective governance in the hands of the warrior class. Its preoccupation with war led to a strong interest in the medical treatment of the armies. This mixture of religious values and practical military demands allowed the development of medicine that, while strongly integrated with religious ideas, was based on a strong empirical tradition of clinical practice and was of great use to the army. Whereas in other cultures of the ancient world the presence of a powerful priestly caste either choked off the development of empirical medicine (Persia, Israel) or reduced it to second-rate status (Egypt, Babylon), neither of these circumstances occurred in India. Instead, a strong tradition of clinical medicine rooted in a hard empiricism emerged.[8]

Knowledge of military practice in India in this period is fragmentary.[9] The Aryan invaders introduced the horse and chariot to Indian warfare against the indigenous peoples of the region. The chariot offered an enormous advantage against a people barely out of the Stone Age, and the Aryans were able to establish their dominance on the plains of the Indus quickly, driving the original peoples into the jungles and forests. Aryan infantry depended heavily upon the bow, but it was also equipped with bronze swords and axs. A portrayal of Ravana, the monster king of Ceylon, shows him equipped with the weapons typical of the armies of the Brahminic period: dagger ax, club, mace, lasso, trident spear, crescent ax, cane arrow, incendiary arrow, leaf-point javelin, iron-tipped spear, sickle-sword, sword, battle ax, trident dagger, and composite bow.[10] Iron weapons did not appear in the region until the fifth century BCE, so the metal used in these weapons was probably bronze or copper.[11] Over time, the chariot gave way to the war elephant and the warhorse as the primary mounts of the warrior aristocracy, with the warhorse being held in almost mystical esteem. By the sixth century BCE, Indian armies had large cavalry contingents.

Little is known about Indian tactics. It appears that the bowmen did not carry shields, but they were protected in battle by a line of shield bearers armed with the javelin. The bowmen and shield bearers also carried broad-bladed swords. While the main tactical idea was to decide the battle by long-range fire from the bow, in cases when this gambit failed, the battle was decided in the usual melee of swordsmen, javelineers, and cavalry in close combat supported by elephants and chariots. Alexander faced this strategy at the battle of the Hydaspes River in 326 BCE.[12] The Indian military physician, then, had to tend the usual array of cuts, bruises, fractures, and penetration wounds that all military physicians had been forced to deal with since the time of Sumer.

Indian Medicine

The highly empirical nature of Indian medicine is what gave it value on the battlefield. This empiricism, however, existed within a strong, overarching religious structure that governed not just medical practice but all things of this world. Yet the doctrinal tension that characterized religion and medicine in other ancient societies did not develop in Indian society. Rather, the physician saw empirical treatment as going hand in hand with religious practices—omens, incantations, psalms, prayer, and so on—as the basis of good medicine. A fundamental assumption of Indian medicine held that the physician must treat the whole person in all his dimensions, including religious ones. The physician usually began medical treatment by consulting omens, engaging in ritual incantations, or saying a prayer over the patient. Having completed this phase, the doctor went on to apply empirical treatments, including surgery. After the treatment, the physician concluded the procedure with more incantations and prayers, stressing as a cardinal rule that the patient's mental state—such as being at one with himself or avoiding certain bad habits—was vitally important to successful healing.

Unlike ancient Hebraic and Assyrian physicians, the Indian doctor regarded clinical practices as a separate element of the overall medical treatment but performed them with as much rigor as the religious element. Unlike Greek physicians who were philosophically against religion, myth, and superstition, the Indian doctor saw no reason to reject religion as antithetical to empiricism. The Indians saw healing as a process that involved all aspects of the patient and thus joined psychology and clinical practice with little difficulty. Modern medicine is only beginning to recover from the tension, inherited from the Greeks, between psychological and empirical aspects of healing and to appreciate the value of the patient's mental state in the recovery process.[13] Meanwhile, the union of the two approaches was a cardinal tenet of ancient Indian medicine.

Indian medicine stressed that recovery from illness was a function of four factors. Of primary importance was the role of the physician in both a religious and empirical sense, and his skill was highly prized. The second component was the quality of the treatment itself, whether involving drugs or surgery, and had to be medically precise and of proven clinical value. Indian medicine stressed the importance of the quality of nursing and posttreatment care, including rest, diet, and changes in behavior, administered to the patient as a third independent factor. The idea that a successful recovery required time and rest from daily rigors represents an important medical advance, one that Greek and Roman physicians later adopted. The final element of successful treatment encouraged the patient to cultivate positive mental states, which involved following religious strictures and even changing the patient's thought processes. The use of the chanted mantra as a means to relax and to engender alternative mental states played an important role. Modern medicine would recognize all of these factors as having a solid empirical base in a successful recovery.[14]

While this analysis emphasizes the clinical tradition in Indian medicine as it relates to the practice of military medicine, two major theoretical orientations of the Indian medical tradition deserve attention. The first was that man's general physiological health depended on four elements within the body remaining in balance: *vata* (wind,) the most powerful and dangerous of elements affecting health; *pitta* (bile); *kapha* (generally translated as cough or phlegm); and *rakta* (blood). As long as these four elements remained in balance, good health was assured.[15] All diseases were regarded as humoral disturbances. This theory strongly resembles the Greek humoral theory that served as the basis of Greek medicine and almost without change was transmitted to the West, where it continued to be used at least until the eighteenth century CE. While it is tempting, as some authorities have done, to suggest that this humoral theory was transmitted to the Greeks through Persian contacts with both cultures, no evidence supports this view. It does seem unlikely that such a central medical concept would have developed in both cultures without some transmission mechanism, but that mechanism is unknown.[16]

The second guiding theoretical principle of Indian medicine designated *marmas* (critical points) in the body that had profound medical effects and set stringent clinical limits on medical treatment. Each marma was associated with a set of empirically verifiable symptoms that resulted when one of these critical anatomical points was damaged. Each marma had its own name, and the medical texts list 107 of them. Over many centuries, Indian physicians used their clinical observations to note the precise effects of wounds to or near each marma. This information permitted them to determine with some regularity the clinical protocol employed for each injury or disease, as well as the prognosis for a successful outcome. These physicians also understood that the prognoses for injuries to certain marma were not very good. In these instances, the doctor's role was to monitor the progress of the injury and verify that its progress matched the clinical prognosis. These practices strongly parallel the chronicling of empirical clinical observations that marked the writings of Hippocrates. Indian physicians were great recorders and classifiers of their clinical experiences, a habit that produced a remarkably large medical nomenclature and vocabulary.[17] Whether the Indian practice of medical classification was transmitted to Greece or whether it developed there independently is not known; however, clearly both the theory of humors and marmas are much older in Indian medicine than in Greek medicine. The idea of marmas as an aid to clinical observation is found in the Rig Veda, a text that dates from between 1500 and 1200 BCE, long before empirical medicine made its appearance in Greece.[18] If one culture transmitted medical knowledge to another, it most certainly ran from the Indians to the Greeks and not the other way around.

Indian understanding of human anatomy generally reflected the same limited anatomical knowledge found in the other medical traditions of the ancient world. Much of this stemmed from the Vedic proscription against touching the dead lest one be defiled, a stricture that prevented dissection.[19] But their working knowledge of anatomy—that is, its clinical applications— was excellent and based on centuries of recorded observation. These empirical observations, codified in the marmas and the medical texts, served to underpin excellent clinical practice albeit one devoid of anatomical accuracy. Medical practice tended toward specialization, as did all medical traditions of the ancient world, but not to the degree found in Egypt. The religious belief that the whole person had to be treated militated against the Egyptian model of extreme overspecialization.

Medicine was not taught in the priests' schools or academies. It was obtained from serving long apprenticeships with practicing physicians, a model used in the West and on the American frontier until the nineteenth century. The approach to medical study was primarily rational, and the medical education was of high quality. A student's acceptance into the profession was marked by a solemn ceremony in which an oath similar to the Hippocratic oath was administered. As part of his medical training, the apprentice had to commit the Veda medical texts to memory and be able to repeat and chant the relevant sections. His extensive education required the memorization of formulas for medical compounds and the entire sum of available experiential knowledge of surgical and medical techniques. Some idea of the difficulty of this task is obtained from the fact that the *Sushruta Samhita* is seventeen hundred pages long and the *Charaka Samhita* is twice as long.

Emphasis was placed on holistic medicine, or on treating the patient with the full range of complementary religious and empirical means available. The role of religion in Indian medical education is reflected in the fact that the *Charaka Samhita* placed religious treatment first. Meanwhile, the *Sushruta Samhita* surgical treatise assigns surgery to the top of the list of medical treatments. Given the amount of medical lore that the apprentice had to learn, it is likely that the medical training of the Indian vaidya was the most rigorous in the ancient world.

An analysis of those Indian empirical techniques most useful to the battle surgeon reveal a level of clinical practice that surpassed that found in classical Greece and, in some other areas, even the medical skills of Roman military physicians. The eight basic surgical techniques available to the military surgeon included incision, excision, scraping, puncturing, probing, provoking secretion, suturing, and removing "foreign bodies" by using various types of probes to determine the exact location of missiles that had penetrated the body. Other treatments included injections with syringes, cautery, chemosurgery with caustic salves, hemostasis, and amputation.[20] Competent surgery was the most brilliant achievement of Indian medicine, and Indian physicians operated for cataracts, removal of bladder stones, tumors, mastitis, scrofulosis, goiter, hydrocele, hemorrhoids, polyps, anal fistulas, and intestinal occlusion.[21] Indian surgeons were particularly proficient in facial reconstruction surgery of the ear and nose, having gained this expertise as a consequence of helping people whose features were mutilated as punishments for breaking the law. Indian surgeons also experimented with anesthetics. Around 1840, James Esdaile, a British surgeon, brought to England the Indians' use of hypnosis as an anesthetic. The idea did not catch on, though, as chemical anesthetics had recently made their appearance in Western medicine.

With such an extensive practice of surgery, it comes as no surprise that Indian doctors were well aware of the dangers of infection and recognized fever as an indication of the disease process. Unlike Greek, Indian medicine did not regard pus production as a natural and beneficial phenomenon; instead, practitioners saw infection and pus consequences of improper technique on the part of the physician.[22] Indian physicians recognized that some types of injuries could be made fatal if the physician operated too closely to the patient's relevant marma. Instructions with regard to cleansing, treating, and bandaging wounds make it clear that the physician's incompetence can cause events to take a fatal turn. There is, for example, a list of no fewer than twenty things that can go wrong with a simple incision if the physician does not take proper care.[23] The idea that the physician himself could cause infection through improper technique was not introduced into Western medicine until well into the nineteenth century. By that time, the germ theory of contagion had replaced the concern over marma.

Attempts to prevent infection are clearly reflected in the detailed instructions for treating wounds properly. There are injunctions to carefully wash wounds prior to further treatment. The *Sushruta Samhita* is clear: no wound should be stitched "as long as the least bit of morbid matter or pus remains inside it."[24] Indian physicians developed a wide variety of forceps with special shapes for extracting foreign matter from battle wounds. No fewer than fifteen different modalities for extracting missiles from wounds are recorded, including the use of magnets to retrieve pieces of iron from the soldier's body.[25] A variety of probes were also used in wound treatment.[26] If carefully followed, the simple practice of thoroughly cleansing wounds would have drastically reduced infection rates, especially for tetanus and gangrene. Once cleansed, wounds were treated with a salve made of honey butter that was essentially the same honey-based ointment that Egyptian physicians used, as noted in the Smith Papyrus. As seen in chapter 4, until the invention of penicillin, honey as a wound dressing was the most powerful bactericidal compound available to medicine.[27] Other wound dressings included ghee, a clarified butter that was aged in special tanks and prepared over long periods specifically as a medicinal compound.

A cleansed and treated wound was sutured with special needles designed for the purpose. Common suturing threads were made of cotton, Chinese silk, hemp, linen, and even horsehair.[28] In suturing wounds of internal organs, such as the intestines, Indian surgeons used the heads and jaws of large ants as clamps.[29] As the wound healed, the ant heads were gradually consumed by the patient's body. It is the first evidence of dissolvable sutures in history.

Wound treatment was complete after following careful instructions on how to apply bandages. Linen and cotton bandages were often tied in the shape of a figure eight (the *svastika*), and the knot was never tied over the wound itself but always above it. Medical texts detail specific instructions for changing bandages. In summer, the bandages were to be changed every day, while in winter they were changed every three days. If a patient was in pain, however, the physician was obliged to examine the wound immediately. Following these procedures, undoubtedly they would have saved the lives of many wounded soldiers.

India was one of the most malarial countries on the planet, as well as a breeding ground for plague and cholera. Not surprising, Indian doctors were acutely aware of the possibility of epidemic, and Indian medicine placed great emphasis on prevention through personal hygiene. Physicians recommended tooth brushing, chewing betel leaves, anointing, combing, exercising, getting massage, regular bathing, and eating proper food as a way of preventing illness. Special instructions were issued during epidemics to avoid fly-infested food, dirty water, and raw vegetables. The effectiveness of Indian medicine is most obvious in that for thousands of years Indian physicians prevented smallpox epidemics by inoculation, a technique the Europeans learned from the Turks only during the eighteenth century.[30]

Indian physicians seem to have been the first to use the tourniquet. The development of the tourniquet resulted from the need to treat snakebites. The bites of deadly poisonous snakes were a serious medical problem for Alexander's troops during his invasion of the Indus Valley. Having found his own physicians helpless to deal with the problem, Alexander commandeered Indian physicians to treat his stricken soldiers. These physicians treated snakebites by tying off the area of the bite with a pressure tourniquet to stop the poison from infecting the body through the bloodstream. Modern experiments show that this technique was effective at stopping venous blood flowing back to the heart.[31] After lancing the wound, the tourniquet allowed arterial blood to flow out of the open wound and cleanse the poison from the body. This use of the tourniquet does not constitute the introduction of the hemostatic tourniquet of later invention; however, its place in the *Sushruta* constitutes the instrument's first documented medical use in history.[32]

Perhaps even more impressive was the remarkable ability of Indian physicians to invent a clinical procedure for surgical amputation. It is amazing to discover this innovative technique in the Indian medical texts. The Vedic texts even record the replacement of amputated limbs with iron prostheses. Greek physicians never mastered amputation and only rarely attempted it. Hippocrates warned against its use as almost always resulting in death. Indian doctors apparently performed amputations with some regularity and were fairly successful at it.[33] It also seems likely that they regularly used wine and other drugs as primitive anesthetics to dull pain during these operations.[34] The massive bleeding that often accompanied these operations was controlled by cautery with a hot iron rod or by immersing the amputated limb stub in hot oil, techniques still commonly used during the American Civil War. It also seems likely that surgeons familiar with the tourniquet in treating snakebites would have eventually stumbled upon its use as a hemostatic device to stem bleeding in amputation.

Indian medicine developed an extensive materia medica of more than six hundred identifiable botanical compounds and over twice as many drugs and medicants as found in the pharmacopoeia of Greek physicians.[35] The stress on botanical compounds instead of the chemical compounds that the Egyptians used seems more in line with the tradition of Babylonian and Assyrian medicine. There is no evidence that Indian doctors used any chemical compounds such as copper sulfate. The Vedic texts mention a class of herbs that were used specifically for treating battle casualties, including *visalya* to stop bleeding and *vishalya karani* for those knocked unconscious.[36]

Indian Military Medicine

The constant warfare among the tribal principalities of the Ganges Valley civilization and the prominent role of aristocratic warrior castes in these wars inevitably engendered a concern for military medicine among the most powerful members of society. This concern is evident from the earliest days of Vedic society. One of the oldest texts, the Rig Veda, written in the mid- to late second millennium BCE, contains accounts of battles, weapons, and wounds and is complete with a list of medical treatments used to treat battle wounds.[37] The early Vedic texts mention the presence of military physicians in war, and Vedic mythology tells the story of the Aswins, celestial physicians who were worshiped by the early Vedics for their skill in providing medical treatment to the wounded on the battlefield.[38] Unlike the medical mythology of ancient Sumer, Babylon, Egypt, Assyria, and Greece—all of which note the presence of godlike physicians who watch over the practice of medicine—only the Vedic god of medicine is identified as a *military* physician.

The importance of war and the central place of military medicine as a formative force in Indian medicine are testified to by the fact that the doctor who specialized in surgery was called the *shalyahara*. With the word *shalya* meaning "arrow" and *hara* meaning "remover," the Vedic term for surgeon clearly demonstrates its military origins.[39] From the earliest times, military physicians regularly accompanied Vedic armies. The Rig Veda indicates that legs were amputated and replaced by iron substitutes, injured eyes were plucked out, and arrow shafts were extracted from the limbs of Aryan warriors.[40]

The concern for military medicine is also evident in other texts. The instructions given by Bhisma to Yudisthira the king were that he had to know not only the methods of warfare but also the diseases and injuries that afflicted his troops. The king was ordered to take proper care and ensure that the means to protect and treat the troops on the battlefield were at hand. Drugs and medicines were to be stockpiled in advance, and surgeons were always to be in attendance.[41] Other texts instructed the commanders of the army to use physicians to inspect campsites and to maintain the cleanliness of the food and water supply.[42] The solid empirical reasons for carrying out these hygienic practices were listed in detail. The *Mahabharata* bids the commander to maintain four types of physicians in his camp, some of which should be expert in treating poisoning cases and others in extracting arrowheads from the body.[43]

Still other texts note that doctors were to attend the army while on the march and that the physician had the responsibility for treating injuries and ensuring a proper food supply.[44] A separate section describes the preventive health measures to maintain the fitness of the army. The *Arthashastra* offers more clues to an effective military medical service. It describes the existence of a military ambulance corps drawn by horses and elephants. The armies were regularly attended by complements of surgeons, and the commander was enjoined to see that sufficient doctors, instruments, drugs, and cloth for bandages were in the baggage train. Also mentioned is the presence of women, who provided food and beverages to the troops and recited encouraging words, in the first evidence of the use of female nurses.[45] The importance of the medical corps is further testified to by the directives that the medical tent be placed near the king's command tent and that a flag be flown from the medical tent so that its location could be easily found, thus minimizing the delay in bringing the wounded to it.[46] Finally, the king was instructed to accompany the physician on regular visits to the wounded and to praise the bravest men, lifting their spirits and aiding their recovery.[47] Nowhere else in the early ancient world is there evidence of a military medical service so organized and so integrated into the military structure as the Indian military medical corps. Indeed, one gets the impression that a great deal of the empirical clinical medicine in the Indian tradition stemmed from the military physicians' efforts to treat the myriad casualties that resulted from the almost endless wars.

A remarkable aspect of the Indian medical corps was the recognized status of physicians and surgeons as noncombatants, a development that did not come about until much later in the West.[48] This status must have been bestowed grudgingly in the ancient world and then only on those professions that were seen to have great value to the military effort. The frequent wars fought by armies of warrior aristocrats led to a code of military chivalry that served to reduce the horror of war. In the "Shanti-parva," for example, soldiers were instructed that they should cease fighting if their opponent became disabled. Moreover, a weak or wounded man should not be slain. Any warrior who threw down his weapons and pleaded for his life should also be spared. A wounded soldier should either be sent home or, if brought to the victor's tent as a prisoner, should have his wound attended by military physicians. Further injunctions prohibited killing those who were weakened by thirst and fatigue or who had been driven insane. Camp followers were also to be spared.[49] The recognized role of the physician in ethically enforcing these edicts presaged his role in modern times by almost two thousand years.

The *Sushruta Samhita* has already been mentioned as a masterpiece of surgical knowledge. The fact that many of its clinical descriptions address the injuries that would be routinely encountered on the battlefield lends credence to the idea that military medicine helped spur the development of the general Indian medical tradition. The *Sushruta Samhita* addresses a full chapter to surgical appliances, bandages, dressings, and medicinal plasters that had primary military applications.[50] One section on belly wounds is brutally graphic. Here the author describes what to do when the patient's belly has been ripped open and his intestines have spilled upon the ground. The author explains a procedure for replacing the slippery coils back into the body cavity. If the intestines have been exposed too long and have dried, the physician is to first wash them in milk and then lubricate them with ghee before replacing the intestines. If the intestines are perforated, the tears must be sewn before being returned to the body cavity.[51] The author seems to be dealing with the kinds of belly wounds found only on the battlefield, and the description is far too accurate not to have been recorded by a physician who had direct experience with this type of wound—in short, a military surgeon.

Nowhere in the early ancient world does one encounter a medical tradition that was more empirically and pragmatically oriented than the Indian tradition. It far surpasses anything that came before it, and in most major aspects—its empirical description of clinical conditions, treatment of infection, surgical skill, hemostasis, drugs, and amputation—surpassed any level of medical development until the time of Rome. No military medical service of the ancient world except Rome's surpassed that of the Indian armies. The close integration of the medical profession within the military forces of the day represented a major advance in military medicine, as did the status of physicians as noncombatants and the accompanying codes of behavior that limited the killing of the enemy and dictated doctors' care for the enemy wounded.

Most impressive was the manner in which Indian physicians fit their professional status and the empirical practice of medicine and surgery into the larger religious context of Indian society without sacrificing the effectiveness of their clinical practice. For most of the societies of the ancient world, this pragmatic compromise of religion and medicine never occurred. The general result was that elsewhere, medical discovery, experimentation, and clinical practice remained at much lower levels than in Indian society. Since no evidence shows that any of the clinical knowledge of Ayurvedic medicine ever found its way to the West through cultural transfer, perhaps the most enduring legacy of the Indian vaidya is the idea, evident in the West only after the Renaissance, that religion and medicine can live well together as long as the central focus of both rests on the inherent value of the human being as he is found on this earth rather than as he will be found in some afterlife.

Notes

1. See Erwin H. Ackerknecht, *A Short History of Medicine*, rev. ed. (Baltimore: Johns Hopkins University Press, 1982), 35. Ackerknecht notes that "although the ancient civilizations have died out, the Oriental civilizations of the river valleys of India have survived up to the present time. And their systems of medicine have survived with them. Thousands of practitioners still apply these ancient types of medicine to millions of patients." See also Prakash N. Desai, *Health and Medicine in the Hindu Tradition: Continuity and Cohesion* (New York: Crossroads Press, 1989).

2. Majno, *Healing Hand*, 261.

3. Ibid., 262.

4. For an account of warfare in the Indian states, see Gabriel, *Empires at War*, vol. 1, *From Sumer to the Persian Empire*, chapter 9, "India."

5. The basic sources for information on Indian medicine include H. R. Zimmer, *Hindu Medicine*, ed. Ludwig Edelstein (Baltimore: Johns Hopkins University Press, 1948); Garrison, *Notes on the History of Military Medicine*, 33–35; K. K. Bhishagratna, trans. *Susruta Samhita*, 3 vols. (Calcutta, 1907); the *Charaka-Samhita,* trans. Avinash Chandra Kaviratna, Calcutta; Ackerknecht, *A Short History of Medicine*, chapter 4; Majno, *Healing Hand*, 259–68; B. V. Subbarayappa, ed., "Medicine and Life Sciences in India," in *Fundamental Indian Ideas of Physics, Chemistry, Life Sciences, and Medicine,* vol. 4 of *History of Science, Philosophy and Culture in Indian Civilization* (New Delhi: Munshiram Manoharlal Publishers, 2002), part 2; A. M. Acharya, "Military Medicine in Ancient India," *Bulletin of the Indian Institute of History of Medicine* 6 (1963): 51–57; U. P. Thapliyal, "Military Organization in the Ancient Period," in *Historical Perspectives of Warfare in India: Some Morale and Materiel Determinants*, ed. S. N. Prasad (New Delhi: Centre for Studies in Civilizations, 2002), vol. 10, part 3, 91–93, for the medical service; Dorothea Chaplin, *Some Aspects of Hindu Medical Treatment* (London: Luzac, 1930); and Abdur Rahman et al., *Science and Technology in Medieval India: A Bibliography of Source Materials in Sanskrit, Arabic, and Persian* (New Delhi: Indian Natural Sciences Academy, 1982).

6. Majno, *Healing Hand*, 263, puts the date of the written treatises at 400 CE while Ackerknecht, *Short History of Medicine*, 36, puts the date at 800 to 1000 CE.

7. Majno, *Healing Hand*, 264.

8. The tension between religion and medicine reappears in almost all ages of history and persists today, for example, in the debate over stem cell research and when life itself begins. The propensity for organized religious groups to define questions of fact from religious dogmas seems as old as humankind itself. For more on this tension, see Mildred E. Mathias, "Magic, Myth, and Medicine," *Economic Botany* 48, no. 1 (January–March 1994): 3–7.

9. Gabriel, *Empires at War*, vol. 1, chapter 9; and Thapliyal, "Military Organization in the Ancient Period."

10. Gabriel, *Empires at War*, 1:239.

11. Dupuy and Dupuy, *Encyclopedia of Military History*, 12–13, 35. The Indians did develop a process for making iron, but they never seemed to have been able to make it in any quantity.

12. Ibid., 35.

13. For more on this holistic approach as it applied to ancient medicine, see Gabriel and Metz, *From Sumer to Rome*, chapter 7.

14. Ackerknecht, *Short History of Medicine*, 40.

15. Ibid., 37; and Majno, *Healing Hand*, 276.

16. Regarding this humoral theory, both Achayra in "Military Medicine in Ancient India" and Dehesh in "Pre-Islamic Medicine in Persia" suggest a case for cultural transfer through Persia to Greece.

17. Ackerknecht, *Short History of Medicine*, 39.

18. Majno, *Healing Hand*, 278.

19. The *Sushruta Samhita* recommends an alternative process. Submerge a cadaver in a pool of water for a week until putrification sets in. Using a pole, the physician can then pull the flesh off the body, revealing its inner organs without having to touch the corpse itself.

20. Ackerknecht, *Short History of Medicine*, 41.

21. Ibid.

22. Majno, *Healing Hand*, 287. The Greek doctrine of "good pus" passed unchanged into Western medical practice and probably caused more deaths than any other medical practice until the nineteenth century.

23. Ibid.

24. Ibid.

25. Ackerknecht, *Short History of Medicine*, 41.

26. Indian medical texts describe 120 various surgical instruments. Garrison, *Introduction to the History of Medicine*, 34.

27. Gabriel and Metz, *From Sumer to Rome*, chapter 7.

28. Majno, *Healing Hand*, 302. During the Civil War, the Union blockade deprived Southern physicians of silk for use as sutures. Southern doctors turned to horsehair as suture material. To make the horsehair flexible for use, it had first to be boiled in water, which also made the horsehair sutures sterile, something that silk thread was not. One consequence was that the South had fewer cases of wound infection than the North had.

29. Ackerknecht, *Short History of Medicine*, 41.

30. Ibid., 42.

31. Majno, *Healing Hand*, 283.

32. Ibid.
33. Ibid., 311.
34. Ibid., 295.
35. Ibid., 311.
36. Thapliyal, "Military Organization in the Ancient Period," 93.
37. Acharya, "Military Medicine in Ancient India," 50. This is the only source that attempts to describe the ancient Indian military medical system in detail.
38. Ibid., 50–51.
39. Thapliyal, "Military Organization in the Ancient Period," 92.
40. Ibid.
41. Acharya, "Military Medicine in Ancient India," 52.
42. Ibid.
43. Thapliyal, "Military Organization in the Ancient Period," 93.
44. Acharya, "Military Medicine in Ancient India," 52.
45. Thapliyal, "Military Organization in the Ancient, Period," 93.
46. Acharya, "Military Medicine in Ancient India," 54.
47. Ibid.
48. The Geneva Convention of 1920 promulgated the official recognition of the noncombatant status of physicians in war.
49. Acharya, "Military Medicine in Ancient India," 52.
50. Ibid.
51. The description of the procedure appears in Majno, *Healing Hand*, 304.

8

GREECE, 500–147 BCE

This is a good place to remind the reader that the development of medicine as a cultural achievement of the civilizations of the ancient world did not occur in any systematic manner that can be attributed to ancient civilization as a whole. Medicine developed almost uniquely within the confines of each separate culture, with little in the way of knowledge transfer from one culture to another. Even in those ancient societies that coexisted, the degree of transfer of medical knowledge, where it happened at all, tended to be remarkably small. In other instances, when the empires collapsed, whole traditions and bodies of medical knowledge were completely lost without any information passed on to the rulers of the succeeding empires. Thus, the long, written clinical tradition of Assyrian medical pragmatism died with that empire and deprived the Persians and Greeks of any benefit that might have accrued from it. The predominant cultural biases of a given ancient civilization so strongly shaped each separate medical tradition as to present almost insurmountable barriers to the transfer of medical knowledge from one age to the next. One major exception was Greek medicine, which had a significant impact on Roman medicine and, ultimately, on the general medical tradition of the West.

Greek Medicine

Western medical histories often portray the Greeks as the "fathers of modern empirical medicine." This claim is based on three fortuitous events, none of which involved the quality of Greek medical knowledge or practice per se. First, of the major ancient civilizations, the Greeks were the first to write in a language that the entire population of their culture as well as foreigners could understand. This written language was distinct from the ideographic-phonetic cuneiform and hieroglyphics of previous cultures that were used only as administrative languages. The availability of common writing ensured a much wider distribution of written information than had previously been possible. Second, Greek literature's importance rests in the fact that more so than any other ancient civilization, much of it had the good fortune to survive for analysis by later generations. Third, the incorporation of Greece into the Roman imperium assured that for almost seven hundred years, Greek medical thought and practice received wider dissemination than any other medical tradition of the ancient world, a circumstance that secured its place at the roots of Western medicine. The result of these factors was the idealization of many aspects of Greek culture, including medicine, as a sort of golden age in which clinical medical practice occurred for the first time. The corollary assumption was that Greek medical skills had reached some sort of pinnacle of accomplishment not seen before in the ancient world.

Greek medicine can be correctly regarded only as the major source of *Western European* medicine, however, and only because when compared to Sumer, Egypt, Assyria, and India, Western Europe's lower state of general social development had not produced a medical tradition of any value before that of the Greeks appeared. Viewed in this context, the Greek theory and practice of medicine was, in most respects, *less* advanced than that of numerous earlier civilizations of the Middle East and Asia. Moreover, many medical innovations commonly attributed to the Greeks were already long established clinical practices in the medical traditions of previous ancient cultures. Among these "innovations" associated with the Greeks are the mystic power of numbers in the progress of disease (Babylon, Israel, Assyria); a code of medical ethics and behavior (Sumer, Babylon, India); the dignity of the medical profession as a separate social order (all ancient cultures placed their priest-physicians at a high-level status); the use of the pulse in diagnosis and prognosis (Egypt, Assyria); the recording of surgical procedures (almost all ancient cultures that could write); decompressive trephining (a medical practice since Neolithic times); treating and preventing infection (all except Persia and Israel); wound washing (Sumer, Egypt, India); bandaging (Egypt, India, and others); suturing (Egypt, India); and hemostasis (Egypt, India). At most the Greeks can be said to have reinvented them and, most important, transmitted them into the corpus of Western medical knowledge.

Greek medicine can be divided into two developmental phases: pre-classical medicine (1200–550 BCE) and classical medicine (550–136 BCE). The Alexandrian period is included in the later category, when Greek medical empiricism reached its height and entered the larger scientific world beyond Greece proper. The two periods closely correspond to medicine as magic and medicine as science, although even in the pre-classical period there are examples of pragmatic medicine that are mostly confined to military medicine. And it is beyond doubt that after Hippocrates's era, Greek medicine still contained a strong element of pre-classical mysticism and magic that coexisted alongside the empirical school, retaining both its status and clientele. Before the Roman occupation, there probably was never a period in Greek history when people visited physicians for help more than they relied upon witches and sorcerers.[1]

Pre-classical Greek medicine, like the early medicine of Sumer and Egypt, was closely associated with magic and religion. The Greeks arrived at the idea, common to all ancient peoples in the early stages of development, that disease and illness were visited upon sinful humans by angry gods. Apollo cast plagues and epidemics upon humans as punishment or signs of displeasure, but Apollo also cured those he struck down. Like other earlier peoples, the Greeks developed the idea that humans could placate the gods' anger through ritual and sacrifice, and these practices formed the center of early Greek religion and medicine. Medicine during this phase was almost entirely prognostic and prophylactic in approach insofar as it was intended to avert or cure disease by ritual sacrifice, including human sacrifice; rites of placation and atonement; and purifying rituals.[2] In all its important respects, the development of early Greek medicine was remarkably similar to that found in the earlier stages of other ancient cultures.

Glimmers of empiricism emerged, however, especially in the practice of military medicine. The importance of warfare in spurring the development of clinical pragmatism in early Greek medicine is revealed in the fact that the old Ionian word for physician, *iatros*, meant an "extractor of arrows."[3] The Hindu word for physician had a similar meaning, one that reflected early Indian history's state of almost constant warfare, which also greatly affected the development of medicine in India. The attachment of Greek physicians to the early religious priesthood was never as complete as it was in Egypt but never so separate as it was in Sumer or Assyria. Greek medicine's attachment to religion remained formal and intrinsic in times of peace, but in times of war when clinical practice was at a premium, it was a different issue. It was precisely the medical realities of the battlefield that initially engendered and then much later sustained the clinical aspects of pre-classical medicine.

The evidence that war stimulated empirical medical pragmatism is clear in the *Iliad*, where both regular physicians and well-experienced warrior chieftains administer medical treatment. Homer's noting that two sons of Aesculapius, Machaon and Podalirius, were commanders of ships and "good physicians both" was the first mention in Greek history of physicians being present with a Greek military force.[4] Throughout the *Iliad* are examples of physicians treating the wounded, who are usually dragged from the battlefield by their compatriots, placed aboard a chariot, and taken to the rear to be treated in medical huts. While Homer cites examples of physicians using songs, spells, and incantations to heal the wounded, there are more instances of physicians attempting clinical treatments. A typical clinical picture emerges of a physician calming a wounded soldier by giving him a drink of wine, loosening the soldier's clothing in the area of the wound, washing the wound with warm water, and then examining the wound. He describes spear and arrow points being withdrawn from the body by widening the wound, followed by treatment with "pain relieving herbs" or the application of the juice of some "bitter root," and bandaging the wound with a woolen cloth. In one instance, Machaon sucked blood out of the wound after extracting an arrow from Menelaus's leg, a practice that survived down to the "woundsuckers" who attended duelists in the eighteenth century.[5] As in earlier cultures, war stimulated the development of clinical techniques to deal with the wounded and played a strong role in early Greek medicine.

For the most part, however, magic and sorcery remained the predominant mode of pre-classical medical treatment and retarded the development of surgery and of a useful Greek materia medica. Greek pharmacology of the period was medically useless, consisting mostly of esoteric sacred potions whose value lay in appeasing the gods.[6] The tradition of magic was tempered, however slightly, by commonsense clinical treatments derived from the inventiveness of physicians and soldiers confronted with the cruel reality of war injuries. The medical tradition remained oral, and medical training was informal when it existed at all. No written medical texts date from this period.

As Greek society gradually recovered from the dark ages that followed the collapse of the archaic Greek civilization, the conditions that sustained a purely magico-religious medicine began to erode. As a consequence of developments in philosophy, by the sixth century BCE Greek thinkers of the Ionian Peninsula began to experiment with the systematic use of the mind linked to empirical observation and explanation. It is an interesting, if inexplicable, fact that most of the best minds of the classical period, including all of Greece's great physicians, seem to have come from the coastal colonies of Ionia or its outlying islands and not from the city-states of mainland Greece. The period's major schools of medical thought were all outside the Greek mainland at Cos, Crotona, Sicily, Rhodes, and Cyrene.[7] The period of Greek classical thinking was marked by its systematic emphasis on empirical observation. This focus is said to have originated with Thales of Miletus (639–544 BCE) and his successful prediction of an eclipse by "listening to my mind." Emerging was the revolutionary Greek idea, forever after the underpinning of Western intellectual history, that it was possible to understand the world through rational applications of reason and empirical evidence rather than with magic and religion. This new perspective placed a premium on observation and systematic thought, first in philosophy, then in science, and then in every discipline. This approach to learning constituted the beginnings of a new epistemology of knowledge that represented a direct challenge to the way pre-classical Greeks explained the world.[8]

While the debate over which rational perspective was to be used to the most benefit continued for centuries, the novel idea of using evidence, investigation, observation, and systematic rules of thinking (logic) to explain the world and guide one's actions set the stage for the emergence of the more clinical practice of medicine in Greece. Whereas in the pre-classical period medicine was seen as an integral branch of religion, medical thinking in the classical era became an integral branch of natural philosophy. This shift put in place the foundation for the establishment of an early science of medicine based on clinical observation and experiment.

The contribution of the most famous Greek physician, Hippocrates of Cos (460–370 BCE), rested more in his method than in his medical innovations.[9] His crystallization of Greek empirical medical practice into the *Corpus Hippocraticum*, a canon of some sixty books on various medical subjects, succeeded in raising Greek medical practice to new social and ethical standards.[10] More significant, however, was his methodological insistence that medical theory and practice be based upon clinical observations, and he rooted medical practice in clinical applications that supported what he believed to be the natural tendency of the body to cure itself.[11] Hippocrates was the first Greek physician to base his medical diagnoses on a systematic and empirical set of observable conditions, including the patient's facial appearance, pulse, temperature, respiration, excreta, sputum, and body movements.[12] This practice remains the basis of medical diagnosis to this day. It is worth noting, however, that every one of the clinical indicators that Hippocrates employed was used similarly, at one time or another, by physicians of earlier medical traditions. Empiricism was new to the Greeks but not to the ancient world.

Hippocrates by no means dominated Greek medicine during his lifetime. Indeed, it is fair to say that empiricism did not influence the everyday world of Greek society at all. Any advances in systematic thinking remained confined to a small circle of society, itself afloat upon a small segment of freemen atop a society of slaves and resident aliens. Moreover, Greek thinkers seemed to have a particular proclivity for pure thought as opposed to applied science, and few philosophers and scientists during the classical period ventured into the world of applied pragmatism. Archimedes, the great engineer, tinkered with mechanics for his own amusement and devised the famous screw for lifting water. But when he was asked to write a handbook on engineering, he refused: "He looked upon the work of the engineer and every art that ministers to the needs of life as ignoble and vulgar."[13] Greek physicians were regarded as craftsmen engaged in physical labor and did not hold high status in Greek society. Unless hired by a city as its doctor, the Greek physician was forced into a peripatetic existence, traveling from place to place in search of paying patients. This wandering effectively precluded the rise of medical schools. The Greek physician learned his trade as an apprentice to his master. Since a reputation for failure was likely to affect his financial opportunities, the Greek physician stressed prognosis over diagnosis, an emphasis that weakened the quality of Greek empirical observation. Physicians often refused to treat cases that were difficult or unlikely to recover in order to avoid the stigma of failure.[14]

The technical base of Greek society was decidedly primitive compared with the great empires of Babylon, Assyria, and Egypt. The failure of the Greek city-states to achieve any sort of central political authority that could direct resources on a large scale meant that in many areas Greek technology lagged behind that of earlier cultures on a state-by-state basis. One beneficial consequence of this political fragmentation, however, was that it prevented the development of a powerful priesthood that controlled medical thought and practice. But linking medicine to natural philosophy contained a fatal trap. The worship of natural processes deduced within the mind or assumed to be true because they were "self-evident" proved to be no less restrictive of empirical observation than religion had been. Facts that did not fit with philosophical premises were rejected or ignored. For the most part, the insular nature of traditional Greek society was not structured to support any type of truly independent empiricism. By the end of the classical period, the clinical approach to medicine had collapsed and mysticism triumphed.

Nonetheless, the Hippocratic methodology was a genuine beginning in medical advancement. With the expansion of Greece into the full-blown Hellenistic phase of its culture under Alexander the Great and his Successors, others adopted the Hippocratic methodology, which came to embody the most important element in Greek medicine for four hundred years. Hippocrates's legacy was the introduction of empirical and pragmatic medicine that spurred the development of the Alexandrian school of medical empirics founded in 331 BCE. In the cultural melting pot of the great Oriental city of Alexandria in Egypt, Greek science produced some of its major achievements at the same time that, paradoxically, Oriental mysticism gained greater influence on Greek thinking.[15] The Empirics were the first Greek medical researchers, and at the school in Alexandria they were driven by the premises that extant anatomical observations were empirically inadequate and required more clinical study.[16] A few of the contributions of the Empirics of Alexandria clearly show how the practice of medicine had become separated from religion. The Alexandrian school practiced the first medical dissections in Greek history, leading to the physiology of the nervous system, the brain, and spinal cord, and distinguished the sensory from the motor nerves.[17] The Greek view of pharmacy changed as well, with a new emphasis on the value of salves and ointments, a development that received considerable direction from Greek contacts with Egyptian physicians. This new view of the medical universe inevitably influenced the pragmatism of medical treatments that were applied on the battlefield.

Greek Military Medicine

It was common practice for the armies of classical Greece to have civilian physicians accompany them in war.[18] Homer's *Iliad* mentions the presence of physicians but not that of priest-physicians. Homer's physicians are all independent craftsmen.[19] Well after the *Iliad*, Xenophon mentions the presence of physicians in the Spartan army and recorded that eight army surgeons accompanied the expedition of the Ten Thousand into Persia at the end of the fifth century BCE.[20] Xenophon tells us in the *Anabasis* that these physicians treated his troops for frostbite, snow blindness, sickness, and gangrenous wounds suffered on the long retreat to Greece after the battle of Cunaxa.[21] He also tells us that some men were assigned to carry the wounded and others hauled the weapons of the men who bore the wounded. But Xenophon mentioned medical services to the troops only once, demonstrating that Greek armies had no regular medical corps even at this late date.[22]

The presence of physicians in Greek armies does not signal the emergence of the first military medical corps in the West. It simply demonstrates the nature of the citizen armies of the period. For the entire classical period, Greek armies remained considerably less organizationally developed than were earlier armies of the ancient world in almost all important respects.[23] Greek armies were small part-time militias raised by each city-state, required little tactical training to implement the simple battle tactics of the day, had no logistics trains or staff organizations, and were incapable of maintaining themselves in the field for extended periods.[24] As such, it is not surprising that they also had no formalized medical support.

The absence of such medical support should not be taken to mean that Greek armies lacked physicians or failed to practice at least rudimentary field hygiene. Homer mentions in *The Odyssey* a kind of "garbage man" who collected human waste and disposed of it outside the camp. Like the Hindus, the Greeks placed great emphasis on personal hygiene, and their goddess, Hygeia, the daughter of the god of healing, was dedicated to cleanliness. There are only a few recorded instances of disease ravaging a Greek military camp in the classical period, and Xenophon advised that military camps be constructed on what he called "healthy ground," that is, at some distance from swamps. It is probably a fair conclusion that Greek armies in the classical period practiced routine field hygiene, a practice made easier by the fact that the armies rarely remained in the field or camp for more than a few days at a time.

While physicians were present on the battlefield, the medical profession remained a private civilian enterprise, and individual physicians sometimes accompanied the army on campaign as a duty of individual citizenship. The physicians' presence was as common as that of other elements of the civilian population—attendants, relatives, wives, girlfriends, prostitutes, merchants, barbers, and others—that accompanied the army. None of these "professions" fell under military law or discipline, and none represented a resource that could be used in a regular manner by the military commander.

Alexander's contribution to military medicine, while still limited, was somewhat more significant, and he seems to have continued the medical support that Philip II of Macedonia introduced. In each instance when Philip was wounded in the field, it is significant that a physician was always readily available to treat him. Unlike the militia armies of the city-states, the armies of Philip and Alexander comprised professionals who served on campaign for months and years on end. It is curious, however, that even during the long campaigns of the Peloponnesian War, Greek armies still did not develop standing medical services. The presence of medical services in Alexander's army was a much more integral part of the army than it had ever been before in Greece. The names of seven military surgeons are recorded as accompanying Alexander on his initial campaign in the East, and records indicate his doctors attended the wounded at the battles of Issus, Zariaspa, and Opis.[25] The presence of physicians at Alexander's death, probably from malaria, is also recorded. It seems clear, then, that Alexander recognized the importance of medical treatment for his troops, especially in his army of professionals, whose losses could not be readily replaced by conscription. He made it a practice to recruit or dragoon whatever physicians came to hand in the captured populations, and he enlisted Indian doctors in the Indus campaign to cure his soldiers of snakebites.[26] Indian medicine at this time was also quite proficient in plastic surgery of the face and nose, especially rhinoplasty. Given the Greeks' cultural emphasis on physical beauty, it is little wonder that Alexander thought Indian physicians valuable.

Alexander also made special provisions for the use of wagons to act as ambulances, again continuing a practice Philip first employed.[27] This accommodation testifies to the value he placed on medical care, for wagons were kept to a minimum in the logistics train to increase the army's speed and mobility and any extra wagons were normally restricted to hauling artillery pieces. While it would be going too far to suggest that Alexander developed the first military medical corps in the West, it is a fair assumption that some of his physicians served for the same long periods of duty that his troops did. Whether these physicians began as military doctors, their long clinical experience on campaign certainly made them practicing military medical professionals in every sense of the word. It would probably be correct to regard Alexander's physicians as the first true military medical professionals in a Western army.

Whatever the quality of Alexander's medical support, it still did not constitute a military medical service. The training of physicians remained a private civilian enterprise, and the army assumed no responsibility for it. Nor did the army make any attempt to ensure that an adequate number of physicians was available. Records indicate the number of doctors attending various Greek armies of the period was relatively small and clearly insufficient for any anticipated medical burden that the physicians would have to face. Xenophon noted eight doctors for his force of ten thousand, while Alexander's first campaign had only seven doctors responsible for the health and care of more than forty thousand soldiers. The small number of physicians in Greek armies suggests that even during the Alexandrian period, medical care may have been limited to high-ranking officers who probably brought physicians along as their personal attendants and at their own expense. Finally, there is no evidence of any trained field medics, apprentices, or medical assistants who provided rudimentary care until a physician could attend the wounded. On balance, the quality of Greek military medical care was quite low throughout the entire Greek period and generally far less than what was available to the soldiers of some of the earlier armies of the period. On more than one occasion Alexander ordered the slaughter of captured enemy sick and wounded so his army could continue to move, suggesting that military medical care had not reached a level evident in earlier armies of other civilizations.[28]

The presence of Greek physicians with the army on campaign makes it certain, however, that some soldiers received medical treatment for their battle wounds. This point raises the question of how effective this treatment may have been. Scores of case studies in the Hippocratic collection cover war wounds, so it may be safely assumed that the Greeks were fairly good field physicians. They were proficient at setting broken bones and dislocations and were among the first medical cultures to use syringes made of animal bladders attached to small pipes for various procedures.[29] The Greeks used the Egyptians' metal probes, but without any evidence that they were washed between examinations, their effect in reducing infection remains doubtful. The Greek physicians were generally less skilled than Egyptian doctors in dealing with head fractures, and the practice of drilling a hole in the skull, even when no fracture was present, and heating the wound to bring on infection and pus was probably lethal. The first well-documented use of the tin pleural drain was a Greek innovation, however, and improved upon similar techniques found in earlier medical traditions that used reed drains. Experience with chest penetration wounds made by spears and arrows finally convinced the Greeks that it was vital to remove the pus from abscessed chest wounds. But inserting an unsterile drain in the chest and applying heat to speed suppuration were probably not successful in most cases.

The Greek physician's treatment of some wounds was, however, quite good. They noted that round wounds did not heal as well as irregularly shaped wounds and generally took much longer. Greek physicians introduced the practice of changing the shape of the wound to an oval, which increased the chances of successful and complete closure.[30] Greek physicians were the first medical practitioners to attempt the use of the hemostatic tourniquet, and they also recognized the risk of producing gangrene in the tied-off limb.[31] Nonetheless, the tourniquet represented a major advance in treating battle wounds in that its proper use would have prevented shock and stopped massive hemorrhage. Since most soldiers wounded in ancient armies died of blood loss and shock, the tourniquet was one of the most potentially revolutionary medical advances of the ancient world. Unfortunately, as with many innovations of the Greeks in so many areas, theory was not followed by systematic application. Greek physicians never learned how to stop heavy bleeding and never conceived of the arterial clamp, arterial suturing, or ligature, additional devices vital to the successful application of the tourniquet in wound surgery. Having stopped the bleeding with the tourniquet, Greek physicians remained at a loss for what to do next. If the tourniquet was allowed to remain, gangrene invariably set in. If the tourniquet was removed, hemorrhaging killed the patient. These mixed, if predictable results, led to the Greek clinical medical practice to abandon the tourniquet. It reappeared in the hands of Roman military doctors, who invented the arterial clamp and learned how to suture arteries, techniques that led to a radical increase in the rate of casualty survival.[32] After the collapse of the Roman imperium, however, the tourniquet, ligature, arterial clamp, and blood vessel suturing disappeared from Western medical practice. The famous French battle surgeon Ambroise Paré reintroduced the tourniquet and ligature in the sixteenth century CE. Paré is still wrongly credited in a number of medical histories with having invented the tourniquet.

Even granting the Greeks credit for a moderate level of skill in battle surgery, Greek methods for treating wounds failed in three important respects, all of which reduced the probability that a wounded soldier would recover from his injuries. The Greeks' philosophical stress on natural processes led them to regard the onset and presence of infection as an indication that the body was healing itself naturally. It was but a short step to the theoretical premise that wounds healing without infection were not being aided by the body's natural processes and that it was necessary to stimulate infection. It became a common and often fatal practice to aggravate uninfected wounds to produce infection. This Greek theory of "laudable pus" found its way into the medicine of the Middle Ages, largely as a consequence of the rediscovery of Greek medical texts and a mistranslation of Galen of Pergamon's works, and plagued battlefield medicine until at least the nineteenth century, with predictably catastrophic fatal results.[33]

Greek physicians never settled on a technique for bandaging wounds, something that Egyptian and Hindu physicians worked out to a science. The question was whether it was preferable to bandage a wound tightly or loosely. Hippocrates held that tight bandaging produced "dry" wounds, a condition he regarded as a natural state necessary for proper healing.[34] The result was that tightly bandaging wounds became an acceptable Greek clinical practice, but it greatly increased the chances of infection, tetanus, and gangrene. This practice also found its way into military medicine during the Middle Ages, with the same disastrous results.

A third shortcoming of Greek clinical practice in dealing with battle wounds resulted from the Greek physicians' fascination with chemical rather than botanical compounds in wound treatment. As noted, the Greek materia medica was decidedly primitive and remained so throughout most of Greek history. The Greeks' interest in chemicals of all sorts resulted from their increased contact with Egyptian physicians during the Alexandrian age. Some of the more common compounds that Greek military physicians used to treat battle wounds were lead oxide, copper sulfate, copper oxide, and cadmia. None of these compounds are particularly useful as bactericides or bacteriastatics, and some can cause lethal tissue damage when applied to an open wound. Unlike almost all earlier medical cultures of the ancient period, the Greeks never truly succeeded in developing a clinical materia medica that was useful in treating battle injuries. As it happens so often in science, the focus on one line of inquiry—in this case, chemical compounds—retarded research into another, or the usefulness of botanical drugs for wound treatment.

Greek wound washes, meanwhile, were generally good. The most common ingredient used was wine, and the most common antiseptic was vinegar, whose active ingredient is acetic acid. When used in 5 percent strength, vinegar is an excellent antiseptic for E. coli, staphylococci, *Vibro cholerae*, and *E. typhi*—all major causes of wound infection. Wine also acts as a generally effective bacteriostatic and bactericide. Contrary to a popular belief that persisted until modern times, the important ingredient in wine is not alcohol but a subgroup of polyphenols called anthocyanins, the most important of which is oenoside. These chemicals are products of fermentation and, if agitated correctly, produce powerful concentrations of polyphenols. Modern experiments demonstrate that in the proper concentrations, these polyphenols are thirty-three times more powerful as bactericides than the phenols Joseph Lister used in 1865 CE.[35]

On the one hand, unlike the Romans' practice, there is no evidence that the Greeks used special kinds of wine in their wound washes. Moreover, the Greeks' preference for light wines probably reduced the medical value of common wines as wound washes. The production of sufficiently strong polyphenols to be medically valuable as bactericides requires a long fermentation process, something not generally used in producing light or sweet wines. The

Romans, on the other hand, preferred strong red wines fermented to the point of being almost vinegar. This strong wine, *acetum*, was the common drink of the Roman soldier and was provided with his regular rations. Acetum is also high in polyphenols. That Roman military doctors used this type of wine as a wound wash almost exclusively is demonstrated by the fact that the Romans transported casks of acetum to military garrisons duty-free because the wine was classified as medical supplies.[36]

Greek medicine can be credited with few genuine innovations that contributed to clinical medicine. One area of military medical practice that the modern Western world owes exclusively to the Greeks, however, is the first practice of military psychiatry. Though, after the collapse of Rome, military psychiatry totally disappeared from medical thought and practice until its re-emergence as a legitimate medical concern in 1905.

Like the Babylonians before them, the Greeks were well aware of mental illness and were the first culture to practice a sophisticated form of psychiatry.[37] Most important for the history of military medicine, Greek physicians were the first to link psychiatric symptoms to the stress of battle. Greek literature is filled with accounts of soldiers driven mad by their wartime experience. Probably the best known illustration of this phenomenon in Greek literature occurs in Sophocles's famous play as Ajax madly slays sheep in the belief that they were enemy soldiers, but Herodotus recorded the actual symptoms of the first clinical case of psychiatric collapse in battle.[38] Xenophon described the first case of psychosomatically induced illness due to fear of death on the battlefield.[39] While Greek society contributed the myth of military heroism to Western thought, it comes as no surprise that Greek thinkers were acutely aware of the failure of nerve that often afflicted troops in combat.

The widespread use of Aesclepian temples, where patients drank of the "water of forgetfulness" and underwent deep, drug-induced sleep as a form of incubation therapy, represented a modern and sophisticated treatment for psychiatric combat reactions.[40] It was also recommended that veterans suffering from mental problems attend the productions of Greek tragedies as a form of abreaction. These plays were probably useful as a primitive form of psychodrama in which the troubled soldier identified with the tragic hero as a way of reliving and relieving his own guilt feelings. While the Greeks can be credited with inventing psychiatric treatment for soldiers, there is no evidence that

Greek physicians used these techniques in any systematic way to treat military casualties. The first hard evidence of any army regularly caring for psychiatric casualties is found in Rome, where soldiers suffering battle-induced psychiatric problems were cared for in the psychiatric wards of legion hospitals.[41] It was not until the Russo-Japanese War of 1904–1905 that any Western army again attempted to confront the problem of combat psychiatry in a systematic manner, with credit generally going to the Russian army for its invention of the practice in the modern age.[42]

Any assessment of Greek military medicine is forced to conclude that while Greece produced an important methodological direction for medical research and practice by attempting to base its medical conclusions upon empirical observation, its physicians' clinical contributions were mostly marginal when compared to the medical achievements of some of the more ancient civilizations. This assessment is not surprising given that Greek society itself was never as fully developed and organizationally articulated as that of Egypt, Babylon, or Assyria. Moreover, Greece was not heir to any systematic medical tradition. With the exception of Egypt, whose contacts with Greece came only after Egyptian clinical medicine had declined to its low point, Greek medicine was almost totally sui generis. The rich medical traditions of Babylon and Assyria died with the destruction of Ashurbanipal's great library, and the Greeks' extensive contact with the Persian Empire produced no new medical lore because the Persians had none to give.

Whatever medical innovations that individual Greek physicians introduced were never systematically applied throughout the medical profession. Thus, while Athenian medicine may be said to have been largely empirical, medical practice in Thessaly and Macedonia remained in the hands of sorcerers and witches. The extreme stratification of Greek society and the strong social distance between classes, in any case, would have nullified attempts at extending medical knowledge and practice to the lower classes that made up fully two-thirds of the state. The Greek proclivity for citizen militia armies as a natural consequence of the country's fragmentation into rival city-states similarly prevented any systematic application of medical techniques on the battlefield. Any effective system of military medical care requires not only sufficient medical knowledge but also the organizational ability to deliver it on a regular basis. This task, however, was beyond the armies of classical Greece.

The establishment of a genuine military medical service corps had to wait until the Romans brought their organizational skills to the task.

By the end of the Alexandrian age, the ancient world can be said to have produced approximately four thousand years of medical history. In that time and in one place or another, humankind had developed almost all the knowledge and clinical treatment techniques that would have been sufficient to produce a relatively effective procedure for successfully dealing with battle casualties. Given the types of wounds produced most often by weapons propelled by muscle power, successful treatment of the wounded in ancient armies required at least five capabilities: (1) to stop bleeding to prevent death by shock; (2) to extract missiles lodged in the body; (3) to cleanse wounds thoroughly with some sort of effective bactericide and bacteriostatic; (4) to suture or ligature veins and arteries and bandage wounds properly; and (5) to prevent infection, since no method of curing infection was available until the mid-twentieth century. Most of the knowledge to accomplish these steps was already in existence although never found completely in a single culture.

Thus, the simple pressure tourniquet made its appearance in the ancient Hindu culture, while the hemostatic tourniquet was first used and then abandoned in Greece. Missile extraction was an old art, as demonstrated by the very word for physician in both Hindu and the archaic Greek originally meant "arrow extractor." By the Roman era, several successful surgical tools had been invented for extracting arrows and slingshot. It was the Romans who made major use of the hemostatic tourniquet and invented the surgical arterial clamp. Various bandaging techniques, including adhesive bandages and clamp sutures, had been available in ancient Egypt, as had a number of generally effective wound washes, some of which were very effective bactericides. Even the loose bandage technique to prevent infection was known for centuries, although it had been rejected in Greece. By the beginning of the Roman imperium, therefore, the world's stock of medical knowledge and technology was quite sufficient for devising an effective system for treating battle casualties.

What had been missing for most of human history, of course, was an army with the level of organizational skill to systematize military medical care. In this regard, the level of medical knowledge available to ancient battle surgeons remained functionally useless until an army could produce the following organizational structures: (1) a trained core of professional *military* doctors who served full-time with the army as a career; (2) a sufficient number of professional medical paraprofessionals, including combat medics and surgical assistants; (3) an ambulance corps for locating and transporting the wounded to the rear; (4) a system of field hospitals to treat serious casualties close to the battlefield; (5) a system of military hospitals for long-term convalescence; and (6) an adequate logistical system and staff organization to sustain the medical system during peace and war. None of the armies of the ancient world came close to the level of organizational development required to make such a system work until the Roman army.

In a real sense, then, the end of the Alexandrian period saw the West poised on the brink of a medical revolution in which the sum of medical knowledge for treating battle casualties had come into being. But that knowledge remained widely scattered in bits and pieces throughout the known world. No society that remained essentially national in outlook, no matter how militarily successful, could hope to incorporate the world's medical knowledge. To do so required a new secular order, one of worldwide scope and practical bent that would allow it to adopt the best ideas of the various cultures. Constructing this imperium required a level of military organizational skill that ab initio would have been readily capable of incorporating systematized military medical care in the same manner in which it had already coordinated other valuable military tasks. The legions of Rome attained all these achievements.

Notes

1. Basic source materials for early Greek medicine include Henry E. Sigerist, *A History of Medicine,* vol. 2, *Early Greek, Hindu, and Persian Medicine* (New York: Oxford University Press, 1961); James Longrigg, *Greek Medicine: From the Heroic to the Hellenistic Age, a Source Book* (New York: Routledge, 1998); Heinrich Gomperz, "Problems and Method of Early Greek Science," *Journal of the History of Ideas* 4, no. 2 (April 1943): 161–76; and Salazar, *Treatment of War Wounds.*

2. Garrison, *Introduction to the History of Medicine,* 82. An analysis of the connection between Greek medicine, religion, and magic is found in Ludwig Edelstein, "Greek Medicine and Its Relation to Religion and Magic," *Bulletin of the Institute of the History of Medicine* 5, no. 3 (March 1937): 201–46. See also Darrell W. Amundsen, *Medicine, Society, and Faith in the Ancient and Medieval Worlds* (Baltimore: Johns Hopkins University Press, 1995).

3. Garrison, *Notes on the History of Military Medicine,* 37.

4. Garrison, *Introduction to the History of Medicine*, 85.

5. *Iliad*, book 4, 218. On wound sucking, see Robert B. Wagner and Benjamin Slivko, "History of Nonpenetrating Chest Trauma and Its Treatment," *Maryland Medical Journal* 37, no. 4 (April 1988): 297–304.

6. Garrison, *Introduction to the History of Medicine*, 82.

7. Ackerknecht, *A Short History of Medicine*, 50.

8. An epistemology of knowledge comprises the assumptions one makes about how one knows, how one knows one knows, and how one demonstrates what one knows. Since the assumptions of an epistemology of knowledge cannot, in themselves, be demonstrated to be valid, the test of an epistemology is precisely its ability to predict.

9. Garrison, *Introduction to the History of Medicine*, 94.

10. Ackerknecht, *Short History of Medicine*, 55–56. Hippocrates neither wrote nor assembled the collection of works attributed to him. The collection probably comprises notes by students and the works of other physicians familiar with Hippocrates's thinking.

11. There is no such natural tendency. The Greek epistemological assumption about natural tendencies was based on the unproven assumption that "a thing's nature is its end." Accordingly, when an observation revealed a contrary result—that is, a tendency "contrary to nature"—the clinical observation must be ignored in order to sustain the assumption. This intransigence is the fatal trap into which Greek medicine fell.

12. Ackerknecht, *Short History of Medicine*, 58.

13. Chester G. Starr, *A History of the Ancient World* (New York: Oxford University Press, 1974), 430.

14. Ackerknecht, *Short History of Medicine*, 63.

15. Ibid., 65.

16. Starr, *History of the Ancient World*, 430.

17. This was the only period in Greek history when dissection was legal. Ackerknecht, *Short History of Medicine*, 65. And regarding the sensory versus motor nerves, see Garrison, *Introduction to the History of Medicine*, 103. For the major innovations in Greek medicine during this period and their innovators, see Ackerknecht, *Short History of Medicine*, 68–71.

18. While there is considerable literature on Roman military medicine, there are only a few academic sources that address Greek military medicine. These include Christine Salazar, "Die Verwundetenfursorge in Heerlen des grieschischen Altertums," *AGM* 82, no. 1 (1998): 92–97; Salazar, *The Treatment of War Wounds*; Karl Sudhoff, "Aus der Vergangenheit der Verwundetenfursorge," *AGM* 21 (1929): 261–72; Humbert Molière, "Le service de santé militaire chez les Grecs et les Romains," *Lyon Medical* 58 (1888): 402–8; and O. Jacob, "Les

cités Grecques et les blessés de guerre," in *Melanges Gustav Glitz* (Festschrift), II (1932): 461–81.

19. Frölich, *Militärmedicin Homer's*, for a good analysis of wounds and military medicine in the *Iliad*.
20. Xenophon, *Anabasis*, book 5, 3.
21. Ibid., book 4, 5.
22. Ibid., book 3, 4.
23. Under Philip II of Macedonia, however, Greek armies began to catch up with other armies of the period in military sophistication. For Philip's contributions to Greek military practice, see Gabriel, *Philip II of Macedonia*, chapter 3.
24. The strength and weaknesses of Greek armies are explored in detail in Gabriel, *Empires at War*, chapter 10, "Warfare in Classical Greece." For tactical weaknesses, see Matthew, *A Storm of Spears*.
25. Arrian, *Campaigns of Alexander*, 2.7.1; 4.16.6; 5.29.3.
26. Ibid., 8.15.11.
27. Engels, *Alexander the Great*, 16–17.
28. See Arrian, *Campaigns of Alexander*, 5.24.7, for Alexander's slaughter of the sick and wounded at Sangala.
29. Majno, *Healing Hand*, 160.
30. Ibid., 154.
31. Ibid., 152.
32. For the effect of these medical practices on the Roman casualty survival rate, see Gabriel and Metz, *From Sumer to Rome*, chapter 7.
33. The most famous Roman physician of the time was Galen of Pergamon (130–201 CE), who wrote no fewer than a hundred medical treatises. His surviving works fill twenty-two volumes. A great surgeon and dissector (he once dissected an elephant), Galen incorporated the Greek doctrine of laudable pus into his written works, although he rejected it as false. Galen's works survived into the Middle Ages, and the lethal doctrine became accepted medical practice until the nineteenth century. Ackerknecht, *Short History of Medicine*, 72–74. On Galen, see George Sarton, *Galen of Pergamon* (Lawrence: University of Kansas Press, 1954).
34. Majno, *Healing Hand*, 176.
35. Ibid., 87–88.
36. R. Davies, "Some Roman Medicine," *Medical History* 14, no. 4 (January 1970): 105.
37. Other cultures practiced psychiatry. See J. V. Kinnier Wilson, "An Introduction to Babylonian Psychiatry," *Studies in Honor of Benno Landsberger* (Chicago: University of Chicago Press, 1965), 289–98; J. V. Kinnier Wilson, "Mental Diseases of Ancient Mesopotamia," in Brothwell and Sandison, *Diseases in Antiquity*, 723–33. An excellent treatment of general psychiatry in the ancient world is

found in Franz G. Alexander and Sheldon T. Selesnick, *The History of Psychiatry: An Evaluation of Psychiatric Thought and Practice from Prehistoric Times to the Present* (New York: Harper & Row, 1966). For a history of the beginnings of military psychiatry see, Gabriel, *No More Heroes*, 97–100.

38. Some scholars have argued, however, that Homer portrays Odysseus as suffering from psychiatric collapse. *Odyssey* book 8, 83.

39. Gabriel, *No More Heroes*, 97–100.

40. On the Aesclepian temples as psychiatric treatment, see D. Kouretas, "The Oracle of Trophonius: A Kind of Shock Treatment Associated with Sensory Deprivation in Greece," *British Journal of Psychiatry* 113, no. 505 (1979): 1441–46; John Romano, "Temples, Asylums or Hospitals?" *Journal of the National Association of Private Psychiatric Hospitals* 9, no. 4 (Summer 1978): 5–12; and M. G. Papageorgiou, "Incubation as a Form of Psychotherapy in the Care of Patients in Ancient and Modern Greece," *Psychotherapy and Psychosomatics* 26, no. 1 (1975): 35–38.

41. McGrew, *Encyclopedia of Medical History*, 192.

42. For a history of the development of military psychiatry in the West, see Gabriel, *Soviet Military Psychiatry*; and by the same author, *The Painful Field: The Psychiatric Dimension of Modern War* (Westport, CT: Greenwood, 1988).

9

ROME,
753 BCE–478 CE

The development of Roman military medicine cannot be separated from the larger cultural and organizational context within which it reached its zenith between 100 and 400 CE. The development of any sophisticated technology requires a high degree of social and organizational maturation and continuity to provide the opportunity for innovation and the supporting infrastructure upon which the development is premised. In the case of Rome, the predominant Roman cultural value was pragmatism writ large over a greater area of the world for a longer period than any organizational, social, political, economic, or military order in ancient history. More than anything else it was Roman pragmatism, stability, order, and organizational longevity that set the stage for the emergence of a military medical system that far surpassed anything the ancient world had ever seen and produced medical care far superior to anything the soldier received until modern times.

The Roman army was the longest-lived political institution in the West. Begun in the eighth century BCE, the army of Rome survived until 478 CE, the date commonly accepted as marking the empire's collapse in the West. However, the army continued to exist under the direction of the eastern empire of Constantinople, where it survived as the best military force in the world for another thousand years until the capital fell to Muslim armies in 1453 CE. From its inception until its demise, the army of Rome survived for 2,206 years. As a social institution it was unique in the West, and its contribution to the development of military medicine was enormous.

The history of the Roman army begins shortly after the mythical date of 753 BCE, commonly accepted as marking the founding of Rome.[1] The early Roman state was organized around tribes and powerful extended families, and this social order became the foundation of the army. Each tribe and family contributed a certain number of infantry and cavalry soldiers to the army, even then called the *legio*. The strength of the army was about three thousand infantrymen and three hundred cavalry, the latter being composed of the nobility who could afford the necessary horses and equipment. Roman military organization and weaponry of this period were strongly influenced by the Etruscans, who, in turn, were influenced by Etruria's contacts with the Greeks. The same hoplite revolution that produced the weapons, formations, and tactics of the Greek phalanx was largely repeated in Rome.[2]

Having secured independence from their Etruscan overlords around 510 BCE, the Romans established the republic that was to last for five hundred years. In its first four centuries, Rome was at almost constant war against its rivals in Italy, which ultimately ceded to Roman domination the entire country as well as the Mediterranean basin. Throughout this period, the Roman army went through several reorganizations, each in response to the hard lessons learned on the battlefield. Each set of reforms resulted in an army that was more organizationally articulated, developed, and sophisticated than before. By the first century BCE, the Roman army had become the most organizationally sophisticated army, and the world would not see one of that caliber again until World War I.

The most significant period of military reorganization occurred under the leadership of the Roman consul Gaius Marius in 90 BCE. The constant warfare and the emerging burdens of territorial expansion forced Marius to change the basis of military recruitment. The traditional middle-class landowners who had provided the military manpower from the republic's earliest days could no longer meet the expanded requirements of Rome's military efforts. Marius opened the ranks of the army to the propertyless of Rome. Roman citizenship was still required, but after the Social Wars (91–89 BCE), Rome expanded its manpower base by extending citizenship to all Italians. The quality of manpower drawn from the proletariat fell below the hardy peasant stock to which the legions were accustomed. To bring the quality up to standard, Marius introduced new drill, training, weapons, and tactical requirements. In 105 BCE, the training methods used in Roman gladiatorial schools were introduced to the military.[3] The result of these reforms was a tough, disciplined, professional army. The old citizen militia army died a natural death.

The new Roman armies were thoroughly professional and almost mercenary in fighting quality, but they were still made up of Roman citizens. Prior to the Marian reforms, the legions had been assembled on an ad hoc basis. Marius transformed the legion into a permanent organization.[4] For the first time in Roman history, the legions remained assembled in times of peace and war. This permanent military structure was a thoroughly professional military organization, but its social base had changed. Unlike the old legionaries, the new military professionals had no source of income outside the army, or farms to return to once the campaign was finished. With no way to sustain themselves after military service, these tough soldiers became a danger to the republic. Soldiers became more loyal to their commanders, who provided booty and land, than they were to the state. Inevitably, the armies became the military instruments of the political ambitions of their commanders.

Marius's new legions proved equal to the task of combat when he used them to stop the invasion of Italy by Germanic tribes at the battles of Aquae Sextiae (102 BCE) and Vercellae (101 BCE). Gaius Julius Caesar used them to subdue all of Gaul. Unfortunately, he also used them to seize political power, initiating a civil war that resulted in the death of the republic before his assassination in 44 BCE. The struggle for power among several factions degenerated into a fifteen-year civil war that saw the best fighting men the world had ever produced pitted against one another in support of the political ambitions of their rival commanders. The civil war ended at the Battle of Actium (31 BCE) with Augustus's defeat of Mark Antony and ushered in the age of imperial Rome. Rome conferred on its empire a time of unparalleled peace, stability, and development. One of the chief legacies of Roman genius was the development of military medicine to the highest level attained in the ancient world.

Roman Medicine

Roman medicine had very little to recommend it prior to the second century BCE. It consisted of home remedies and folklore that every farmer and soldier was expected to know and apply himself. The earliest Romans attributed disease and illness to the usual causes—sin and angry gods. Not surprising, medical treatment used the familiar remedies of incantations, spells, and propitiating rituals. The pragmatic Romans were quick to perceive that medical practice usually did not produce the desired results, however, and developed a strong suspicion of physicians. They held physicians in generally low esteem, viewing them as mercenary charlatans whose primary goal was to bilk the suffering.[5] The fact that most medical practitioners in Roman society at this time were either foreigners (mostly Greeks) or slaves further hardened the generally negative view of the medical profession. That these slaves sometimes used their medical skills to poison enemies and even their masters hardly served to increase the status of the medical profession.[6]

Two other factors contributed to the general Roman contempt of medicine. First, the Roman virtues of stoicism and endurance led the Romans to regard anyone who cried out for medical attention when confronted with pain and hardship, especially soldiers, as unworthy of respect. Soldiers were expected to endure pain and suffering, even death, with quiet resignation.[7] Second, the Roman view of religion was decidedly different from that found in other ancient cultures, especially the Greek culture, where gods were taken seriously and seen as models. In the Roman culture, the gods were simply too abstract and metaphysical to play an important role in guiding the behavior of people in the real world. This belief is reflected in the fact that the Romans never developed the complex theologies that characterized the religions of other ancient cultures.

The most that can be said of Roman religion was that its ritual practices were seen as a way to bind the citizenry of the state together for larger national purposes. In Sir T. C. Allbutt's view, "Rome starved individual religion by identifying it with the state and by using it as a buttress to the imperial power."[8] Unlike other ancient cultures where the priesthood occupied a strong and independent social position, the Roman priesthood was relegated to secondary status and played little or no part in the development or practice of medicine. The advantage of this state of affairs was that no powerful social force arose to retard medical innovation once the state finally determined that medical practice, especially military medical practice, was necessary.

Roman Military Medicine

Roman military medicine can be separated into two phases—the first beginning with the republic and ending with the establishment of the imperium under Augustus, and the second beginning with the professional armies of the empire under Augustus and lasting until the death of the Western empire in the fifth century CE. Both periods closely paralleled the development of Roman medicine in general. Where in earlier cultures, the civilian religio-medical establishments strongly influenced the development and application of military medical practice, the opposite occurred in Rome. It was military medical practice that proved the major influence in the development of medicine in the larger Roman society.

Military medical care under the republic generally resembled the medical care in the armies of classical Greece. From the earliest days, physicians attended to the medical needs of the highest commanders, who provided physicians at their own expense. Medical care for the troops was the responsibility of the individual soldier, as in the *Iliad,* and soldiers took care of one another as best they could, with some gaining reputations for effective medical care learned through hard experience. Throughout the republican period, battle accounts mention soldiers bandaging and treating their own wounds.[9] This self-care led to a problem in which soldiers applied dressings to nonexistent wounds to escape military duty, a practice that was seen repeatedly throughout military history and even to the present day.[10] By the time of Julius Caesar, however, a rudimentary medical system of combat medics was already in place. During the Gallic Wars, commentators note that the soldier expected someone to come and dress his wounds rather than having to treat himself.[11] Caesar made arrangements for evacuating the wounded in wagons, billeting them in private houses, and sending some of them on convalescent leave.[12] But whatever arrangements were made for medical care of the soldier stemmed from the individual proclivities of the individual commanders. There is no evidence of any formal military structures to provide medical support to the troops on a regular basis. This development would await the transformation of the republican army into an army of genuine professionals, a process that had begun with the Marian reforms and came to fruition under Augustus.

The lack of an established military medical service in these early days should not be taken as a lack of regard, either by their commanders or the Roman state, for the troops' welfare. Roman commanders often showed great concern for their wounded. Livy notes that it was common practice for Roman citizens to open their houses to the wounded and to feed and care for them while attending their wounds.[13] Providing such care was regarded as a civic duty. It was also customary for Roman armies to take their wounded along with them after the battle, whether in the advance or even in retreat. They were horrified at the behavior of the Volscians and Carthaginians, who routinely abandoned their wounded.[14] In a number of instances, Roman commanders refused to press a pursuit to military advantage because they wanted to attend the wounded.[15] Roman commanders recognized that if the soldier was not cared for, he would not fight well, and many commanders put their personal resources at the disposal of the sick and wounded as a way of ensuring their troops' loyalty.[16]

Caesar understood the need for some sort of medical service and undertook a number of steps to deal with the problem of casualties, including stationing physicians with his army. However, the changing nature of the army under Augustus required more systematic and permanent measures. Given the low regard Romans had for physicians, it was first necessary to overcome this deep cultural prejudice and attract to the army's service physicians who had a command of medical knowledge and clinical practice that was superior to the generally low level of medicine practiced by the Romans. Greek physicians had begun to travel to Rome as early as the second century BCE, but the Roman populace did not generally accept them. The first Greek physician to establish a regular practice in Rome was Archagathus (219 BCE). That he was known as *carnifex* (the butcher) for his lethal surgical operations suggests that he probably did little to improve the general image of the medical profession.[17]

By the time of Caesar's death, the lack of military medical care for the army could no longer be ignored. Roman medical knowledge was simply insufficient to the task of good clinical care for the wounded. In addition, the age-old practice of billeting the wounded with Roman citizens that worked well as long as Rome confined its military operations to the Italian homeland was not practical for an army engaged in military operations throughout a far-flung empire. For the army to have adequate facilities for treating its sick and wounded, it would have to construct and staff a medical service with its own personnel who could move with the army and be garrisoned with units stationed abroad. Finally, the professionalization of the army made it imperative that medical facilities be provided if the soldiery was to retain its morale and loyalty.

The destruction of Corinth in 146 BCE that accompanied the final pacification of Greece and began its incorporation into the Roman imperium provided the opportunity for Greek medicine to migrate to Rome. In 90 BCE, Roman citizenship had been conferred on all native Italians, and in 46 BCE, Julius Caesar conferred citizenship on all practitioners of medicine for the express purpose of attracting medical talent to Rome.[18] Although Romans continued to regard other pursuits as more noble than the practice of medicine, physicians of Greek and other nationalities flocked to Rome. The Roman prejudice against physicians gradually subsided, and Romans themselves finally began to enter the medical profession. Yet, while Latins represented the greatest number of military physicians, until the end of the empire, a large number of physicians serving with the Roman army had names that suggest persons of eastern, non-Italian origins.[19]

The proximate cause of the establishment of the Roman medical service was the fifteen-year civil war that followed Caesar's murder and the rise of Augustus. The war produced horrendous casualties, as the best professional armies of the ancient world slaughtered one another in internecine combat. Upon achieving victory, Augustus reduced the army to twenty-five battle-hardened legions distributed throughout the empire, reorganized their staff structures, and created the first truly professional military medical corps in Roman history.[20]

To attract physicians to military service, Augustus conferred upon all physicians the equestrian dignity (*dignitas equestris*), which included the rights of full citizenship, the status of a knight, and the right to wear the knightly ring.[21] As a further attraction to military service, physicians were given the customary land grants and retirement benefits of the career legionary, and a retired military physician was allowed to resume civilian practice exempt from certain taxes and civic duties.[22] The military physician also had special legal rights that allowed him to recover any losses incurred to fraud against him while on active duty (perhaps the world's first medical liability insurance). Attracting an adequate supply of doctors regularly from the various provinces of the empire with sufficient financial and status inducements and excellent retirement programs, the Roman army was able to obtain enough physicians to care for the legions until the end of the empire.

The practice of civilian medicine in Rome attracted little attention, meanwhile, and it was not until 160 CE that the state began to provide medical care for the general population through a system of public hospitals and doctors.[23]

Within the army, however, the Greeks' clinical medical practice caught on quickly, and most of the major innovations in medicine made in the imperial period are attributed to military physicians or men who had once been military physicians.[24] While the general level of civilian medical care remained low, albeit superior to that found in previous periods, pragmatic medicine among military physicians reached new levels of excellence. Moreover, the fact that there were no medical schools or established curricula of training in Rome until the third century suggests that only the Roman army had established systematic medical training programs for its physicians.[25] It was only after the reign of Septimius Severus (193–211 CE) that a state license was required for a civilian to practice medicine.[26] Many civilian doctors remained ignorant of advances in medical treatment commonly known to military surgeons serving in the army medical corps. The Roman penchant for written records, a consequence of having established a thoroughly modern military staff structure, ensured that whatever new knowledge and clinical treatments the army practitioners developed received wide dissemination with the military medical establishment. These military medical manuals standardized medical care for the soldier, but a similar procedure was never achieved in Roman civilian medicine.[27]

Military medical care began with ensuring that only the best and most intelligent physical specimens were recruited into the army.[28] Military doctors at legion posts throughout the empire conducted physical examinations of recruits. Intriguingly, since after the first century CE only 1 percent of the army was recruited from Italians (most of whom entered the Praetorian Guard to be posted in Italy), the army had its pick of the manpower pool, which was larger, more genetically varied, and physically stronger than any available to any army of the ancient world. Once in service, the military medical corps strove to maintain the soldier's health by continuously stressing hygienic practices. The systematic use of sewers; a safe water supply; a varied diet; regular health inspections; preventive medicine (such as mosquito netting); food supply monitoring; cremation of the dead outside the city and camp walls; sanitary public latrines often with flushing, running water; and regular washing and bathing created a healthy environment for the soldier.

The horrendous experience with disease during the civil war led Roman commanders to take excellent precautions against its outbreak in garrisons or on campaign. The medical officer responsible for the health of the legion served on the commander's staff, an indication of his importance to the military effort. So good were the living conditions in the Roman legions that despite long service in wars and other arduous activities, the Roman soldier lived almost five years longer than the average Roman civilian did.[29] His superior diet also had the effect of producing five times fewer cavities than the average citizen experienced.[30]

A great deal of thought went into the design of a legion fort to establish a healthy environment for the troops. Marcus Terentius Varro (116–27 BCE), a Roman architect, developed a theory of contagion that was remarkably similar to Robert Koch's germ theory of the nineteenth century.[31] Roman forts were never located near swamps or standing water. Buildings and streets were designed so rainwater pouring from the roofs into channels helped cleanse the streets. A complex system of drains and sewers ensured sanitation and emptied into rivers or streams well below the watering point for animals. Where it was not possible to drain refuse into a moving waterway, large leach fields were constructed. Latrines were continuously flushed, and sewage was removed far from the fort. Latrines were dug to depths of three meters and covered with wooden tops to prevent sunlight from attracting flies to the waste that would spread disease. Hand basins were provided for washing and sponges for wiping one's self. Each fort had its own bathhouse for providing warm, hot, and cold baths; some even offered steam baths. The army set a high standard of cleanliness for the soldier, his clothes, and equipment, and he was required to shave daily and bathe regularly, even when the soldier was in the field.[32] Troops exercised each morning and went on twenty-mile marches three times a month. Some Roman forts had drill halls so the troops could exercise in inclement weather.[33] A Roman fort was a model of military hygiene.

The great advance of Roman military medicine was its incorporation of a professional medical service for delivering care to the troops into the legion's formal organization, something that the armies of the ancient world had not accomplished in even a rudimentary sense since the demise of the Assyrian empire in the sixth century BCE.[34] While many trained doctors entered military service for limited tours of duty, the spine of the regular medical service was made up of physicians, combat medics, and orderlies who were trained by the army itself from its own manuals and in its own military hospitals.[35] As civilian medical training remained largely unorganized and based on apprenticeship, the military's training of physicians was a major innovation. It was standard Roman practice to refer to all recruits, even trained physicians, as *miles,* signifying that they were soldiers first. Even educated physicians had to undergo the standard training for military medical personnel before being granted the title of *medicus.* No Western army undertook the training of its own physicians again until 1865.[36]

The importance of the military medical corps within the Roman legion is testified to by the fact that provision of medical services was a primary responsibility of the *praefectus castrorum,* or the "camp prefect" and the legion's second in command. He was usually the senior professional officer in the legion and reported directly to the commander. The chief medical officer of the legion was the medicus, of which there were three types, each of different ranks and status. The fewest in number were those who had some prior medical training or were often trained physicians who entered military service for specified periods of duty. These positions normally carried senior noncommissioned officer status. Other medici who served as chief medical officers were career soldiers who received their training in the army and enlisted for long periods. One of these, C. Papirius Aelianus, served on active duty until he died at age eighty-five.[37] It is difficult to accurately assess the relative numbers of each type of chief medical officer, but most of them were career military professionals.

Another type of medical officer of somewhat lower standing was the *medicus ordinarius.* This officer entered the army as a regular soldier and received training from the army itself. He could rise to the rank of centurion and was a medical specialist with sound, practical medical training. Other medical specialists assigned to the legion included doctors who were specialists in a particular form of medicine, such as internists, eye doctors, and urologists.[38] Almost the full spectrum of medical specialties were represented within the military medical corps. Surgeons constituted a special medical specialty and were regarded as the most valuable medical assets. Also in evidence were additional medical personnel, such as the *seplasiarius,* responsible for the supply of medical ointments; the *marsus,* who oversaw the treatment of snake and scorpion stings; and the *optio convalescentium,* in charge of convalescent troops. These army-trained orderlies were similar to modern-day enlisted medical orderlies or physician assistants.

One of the legion's most important medical assets was the special squads of *capsarii* (bandagers who served as combat medics).[39] The army trained its own medics, much as armies do today. Reliefs from Trajan's Column depict these medics tending soldiers' wounds.[40] The capsarii are shown wearing the same combat gear that the soldiers do. Their mission was to reach the wounded quickly as the battle raged, providing them with acute medical care until the soldier could be brought to the field hospital tent for treatment by a trained physician.[41] The legion had designated units of horses, wagons, carriages, and stretcher bearers to evacuate the wounded to field hospitals. By the mid-second century CE, the Roman army comprised about 400,000 regular troops. At a minimum, this number of soldiers required some 600 to 800 doctors, or approximately 10 per legion, to provide adequate medical care.[42]

The idea of providing military medical support as close as possible to the battlefield and having special units of combat medics to get to the wounded quickly represented a significant advance in military medicine. The field hospitals supported by medics and an ambulance corps constituted the first evidence of a major principle of military medicine, the principle of immediacy. Roman doctors also practiced the second principle of modern military medicine, triage, or separating out casualties according to the severity of their wounds and evacuating and treating the most severely wounded first. As a professional army, the legions had invested long hours and considerable money in the soldier's training. The medical corps attempted to salvage and return to duty as many wounded as rapidly as possible. This operation represented the first application of the principle of expectancy, an integral premise of modern military medicine.[43]

The medical service was adequately represented in all military branches, in all combat arms, and at all levels of the army. Every legion and auxiliary unit had their own physicians and staff, and each infantry battalion and cavalry regiment had its own medical officer and staff. Even the irregular units had regularly garrisoned medical personnel assigned to them.[44] The navy also had a regular medical corps, and each ship of the fleet had a doctor and small staff regularly assigned to it.[45] The *cohors vigilium* that served as police and firefighting forces, had four physicians assigned to each unit, and they probably provided medical support for each of the duty shifts in the twenty-four-hour day.[46] While a soldier of the legion usually served out his entire career posted to a single legion, physicians were often transferred among legions.[47] This re-assignment made sense insofar as it allowed the army to shift medical assets from legion to legion to ensure adequate medical support where the need was greatest. Roman military hospitals followed a common design plan, but some legion forts located on the frontier, which were expected to face hostilities, were often larger and more fully staffed.[48]

The Roman medical service also operated its own military hospitals for both short-term and convalescent care, and each legion fort contained a fully staffed hospital. The military hospital system originated in the wars against Greece in the first century BCE. The impossibility of leaving the wounded among a hostile civilian population made their evacuation imperative; how-ever, Roman administrators found that many of the wounded died during transport to hospitals in Italy. Accordingly, Roman military planners created a system of hospitals along the major roads leading to the provinces. As the small strong points and temporary forts grew into permanent facilities over time, the hospitals within them grew larger and more sophisticated. By the imperial period, it was standard practice to include a complete hospital in the plans for all major legion forts. Tents arranged in the shape of a hollow rectangle were used as field hospitals before the permanent forts were built or when the army was on campaign. When permanent facilities were built, the construction fol-lowed this same hollow shape.[49] The *valetudinarium*, or "military hospital," was commanded by a chief medical officer called the *optio valetudinarius,* who reported directly to the legion's second in command who had the staff respon-sibility for medical support. The concept of the military hospital is an entirely Roman idea, apparently without precedent in the ancient world. There is no evidence for military hospitals before the Augustan period (first century CE). As the growth of the empire increased the distances separating military units from Rome and made it impossible to send the sick and wounded home for treatment, the need for camp-based medical facilities arose.[50]

The hospital's physical layout reflected a new level of medical sophistica-tion that was not seen again in the West until modern times. The entrance to the hospital opened into a large hall lit by clerestory windows and used as a clearing center for casualties. Beyond this hall and having only one entrance was the operating theater, also lit by multiple windows. Connected to the theater was a small hearth room containing a beehive oven where instruments

Figure 2. *Roman military hospital in Vetera, Germany (200 CE)*

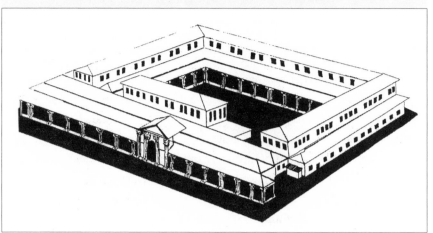

Figure by Tara Badessa

and dressings were sterilized.[51] The hospital kitchen and pantries used to pre-
pare special diets for convalescent soldiers were located on the east side of the
hospital.[52] The western outer wing contained a suite of baths, a dressing room,
and lavatories. The wards occupied three full wings of the building. The ward-
rooms were small cubicles (3.4 by 4.2 meters) arranged in pairs on either side
of a wide corridor, a plan followed typically in hospital construction today.
The entrance to these rooms was through a small side corridor that separated
the rooms themselves from the main corridor to reduce noise and the risk of
infection and contagion. A few of the rooms were reserved for patients who
required isolation. Other rooms were set apart for the hospital staff's use. More
rooms housed examination areas, lavatories, and the hospital mortuary.[53]

The roof of the hospital was constructed in such a way as to provide adequate cooling, ventilation, and fresh air in hot weather, and a central heating
plant ensured adequate warmth in the winter. A central courtyard provided a
source of quiet, fresh air, and light that the wounded could enjoy while con-
valescing. Each legion hospital was constructed to accommodate 6–10 percent
of the legion's 5,000-man strength as casualties, although frontier forts usually
had a larger capacity. In an emergency situation, the reception room, corridors,
and the central courtyard could be used to temporarily house the wounded
awaiting treatment.

The military hospital was among the greatest Roman medical advances, and as with the medical corps itself, there was no civilian equivalent. Unlike other cultures of the ancient world where the advancement of medicine in the military generally lagged behind medical practice in the civilian world, the reverse was true in Rome. Medical science advanced because of the army's systematic organizational approach to medical practice driven by the need to repair and retain casualties in the professional force. As army doctors spread throughout the garrisons of the empire routinely and deliberately searched for new drugs as part of their normal military duties, they expanded the Roman materia medica beyond that of any other in previous cultures. New drugs and other medical information were passed to other medical personnel, often by their incorporation in the army's medical manuals. This method of dissemination allowed medical personnel to transmit a great deal of new medical knowledge throughout the army.

A Roman military physician, Pedanius Dioscorides was the most famous pharmacologist of antiquity. He lived during the first century CE and wrote *De Materia Medica*, the world's largest collection of herbal and chemical medical remedies produced in the ancient world. Written in five books, it was the standard work on pharmacology for more than a millennium and is still read today.[54] The Romans' incorporation of most of the then "known world" into the empire expanded the store of knowledge upon which Roman physicians could draw for new drugs and clinical techniques. Thus, Roman medicine borrowed a number of Indian surgical techniques, including plastic surgery and cataract removal.[55] So many drugs came from India that Pliny complained about it in his writings.[56] In the end, however, Roman medical practice reflected the same practical bent that was such an integral part of the Roman character. Being as closely tied to the military as Roman medical practice was, when the empire collapsed much of the Romans' medical knowledge and clinical technique went with it, lost to future generations for almost a thousand years.

Given the effectiveness of the Roman medical system in quickly reaching the wounded soldier and moving him to a location near the battle where he could be treated by a professional military physician, the question arises as to the quality of Roman clinical medicine and its effectiveness in saving battle casualties. The following analysis is limited to those readily available techniques that the battle surgeon used to deal with combat injury as they appear in the work of Cornelius Celsus, a famous Roman military surgeon. Examined from this perspective, it is fair to say that the quality and effectiveness of Roman military medicine was generally not surpassed until the beginning of the nineteenth century. Celsus lived during the reign of Tiberius (14–37 CE), an early phase of the empire, so the medical practices he records presumably were fairly common at that time and remained so throughout the imperial period.[57] Celsus produced a vast treatise covering the subjects of agriculture, warfare, rhetoric, and medicine. His treatise on medicine, *De Medicina*, comprised eight books. When the empire collapsed, this brilliant and comprehensive medical manual was lost for more than thirteen centuries. It was not rediscovered and reprinted until 1478 CE, when along with Galen's works, it then became a basic medical text for another three hundred years. *De Medicina* is the only Roman medical text to survive in its complete form into modern times.

The first task of the battle surgeon is to stop the bleeding caused by weapons damage and prevent the soldier from dying of blood loss and shock. Developing a surgical technique to cope with bleeding required a much more accurate knowledge of human anatomy than had been available to previous ancient physicians. The Romans had no religious strictures prohibiting dissection, and the large number of criminals, gladiators, and condemned men provided practitioners ready access to cadavers.[58] Consequently, the Romans' understanding of anatomy was far better than any that had gone before. Most important, the Romans recognized that arteries and veins carried blood, not air or other humors as other cultures believed. This basic knowledge of circulatory plumbing allowed Roman physicians to locate blood vessels and deal with severed veins and arteries.[59]

A knowledge of blood circulation would not have been useful without two additional Roman innovations—the hemostatic tourniquet to stem blood flow and a technique to tie off veins and arteries temporarily so they could be sutured. To achieve the latter, the Romans invented the arterial surgical clamp. In addition, they also used ligature, or the twisting of blood vessels into a knot to stem the flow of blood. Roman physicians were expert at suturing wounds, using flax or linen thread. These stitches rotted before the wound was completely healed, so there was no need to remove the stitches. These techniques served extremely well for most battle wounds and had the additional advantage of allowing surgeons to raise amputation to a high art. Celsus was the first to suggest amputation through live tissue, and he used a rasp to smooth the bone prior to closure. Archigenes, who lived under Trajan's rule, was the first to perform amputation by identifying and ligating the major blood vessels *before* completing the amputation.[60] The ability to amputate an infected or gangrenous limb saved a great number of lives.

Roman physicians used a number of drugs as sedatives and painkillers to ease the soldier's pain before and after surgery. They used potions made from the opium poppy and henbane as well as henbane seeds. Henbane contains scopolamine, which is still used as a pre-anesthetic medication today.[61] Dioscorides records the use of white mandrake before surgery, saying, "The doctors make use of this, too, when they are about to treat by cutting and burning."[62] The root of this plant yields hyoscyamine and atropine, both of which are modern surgical drugs.[63] Undoubtedly, mandrake taken in sufficient quantities can produce a degree of unconsciousness to complete a surgical procedure; however, there are risks, as Celsus notes, that "we are afterwards unable to arose the man whom we want to put to sleep."[64] Other analgesics noted in the texts are wild lettuce, anise, sleep nightshade, and various opium potions. These sedatives probably helped somewhat but did not constitute genuine anesthesia in the modern sense. Nowhere in the surviving medical treatises dealing with surgery is there any mention of using anesthesia. It is likely that the available painkillers were administered to relieve the pain of the wound or to relieve the pain associated with postsurgical recuperation. As with all surgery until the introduction of anesthesia in 1846, the surgeon's speed and skill remained critical.[65]

Roman surgical skills were clearly reflected in the number, quality, and innovation of their surgical instruments. The quality of Roman surgical instruments was not surpassed until modern times.[66] The core of the surgeon's *instrumentarium* was the various types of scalpels with replaceable blades that he used in operations. The Romans introduced several new types of surgical forceps, including instruments with ring slides and rifled inner faces that allowed them to be locked in place with one hand. Wound edges were held apart with another modern surgical innovation, the retractor, and wounds were closed with fibulae, or modern surgical clasps that resemble safety pins. An enormous advance to battlefield surgery was the widespread use of an arrow extractor, a kind of hollow spoon that could be slid within the wound along the side of the

Figure 3. *Roman surgical instruments (circa 200 CE)*

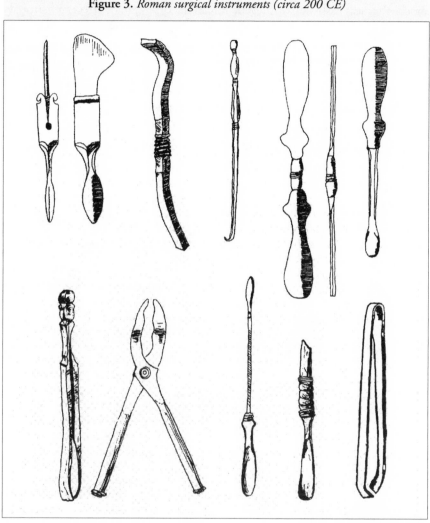

Figure by Tara Badessa

arrow until the arrowhead rested neatly in the spoon for extraction.[67] The Roman surgeon's instruments included far more tools with far more sophisticated functions than any available to surgeons until at least the nineteenth century. As with other aspects of Roman medicine, the collapse of the empire resulted in many of these innovative devices being lost to medical practice for hundreds of years until they were gradually reinvented one by one.

Assuming that a wounded soldier could be saved from blood loss and shock, the next task was to prevent infection. One cannot stress too strongly the importance of preventing postsurgical infection.[68] As late as the mid-nineteenth century, the mortality rate for those operated on in hospitals was often more than one in two.[69] Only after the introduction of antisepsis in 1867 was that figure reduced. The Romans were acutely aware of the danger of infection, and Celsus devoted an entire chapter of *De Medicina* to it. He is also the first physician in ancient history to describe its clinical symptoms and progress in his famous dictum that infection can be recognized by *rubor et tumor cum calore et dolore* (redness and swelling with heat and pain). Perhaps most important in the fight against infection was that Galen's work clearly rejected the lethal theory of laudable pus that had been introduced earlier to Roman medicine. Galen soundly dismissed the idea that infection was a natural part of the healing process when he said, "Those who believe that inflammation necessarily follows a wound show great ignorance. . . ."[70] Roman practice of handling infection was better than the world would see again for more than a thousand years.

It was standard Roman surgical practice to sterilize instruments in hot water before use, a system that again would be not observed in the West until the late nineteenth century. Roman doctors never used the same probe on more than one patient, an important clinical convention that removed the physician as the primary source of hospital contamination. Roman wound washes, especially acetum, were excellent, being more effective than the carbolic acid that Lister would later use.[71] Picking out decayed or foreign matter from a wound before and after repeated cleansing or using maggots to eat the dead flesh (debridement) undoubtedly reduced the rate of tetanus and gangrene, as did the techniques of loose bandaging, surgical clips for closure, drains, and regular changing of dressings. The use of the old Egyptian formula of lint and honey, the most powerful antibacterial potion known until penicillin, to dress wounds was effective, as was the use of *barbarum,* a powerful antiseptic compound that modern experiments has shown to be effective for treating deep flesh wounds.[72]

Roman military doctors would have had a profound effect on the survival rate of the wounded by applying these techniques. Further, Roman medical skill often extended beyond the surgical procedures noted. Plutarch recorded the surgical skill of one Cleanthes, a military surgeon who treated a lower chest wound by replacing the entrails that had spilled out, stopping the hemorrhage, and stitching and bandaging the wound, confident the patient would recover.[73] Celsus explains the procedure for an abdominal operation in which the entrails are spilled, noting that the perforated entrails must be stitched before replacement was attempted.[74] This level of surgery was not attempted again until the seventeenth century.

Roman military medicine in every respect was clearly far superior to that of any other culture of the ancient world and, for that matter, to any military medicine practiced later in the West until modern times. The success of Roman military medicine can be partially attributed to its practitioners possessing the highest level of medical knowledge and skill in the ancient world. But without the organizational genius to design a permanent medical system within the legions that could train physicians and other medical personnel and deliver that care quickly and routinely, Roman medical knowledge would have had far less impact on combat survival rates than it did. Moreover, Roman pragmatism unfettered by religion placed a premium on medical inventiveness. With little in the way of religious strictures to hinder medical investigation, the emphasis fell naturally on what worked. The Romans have to their credit a number of medical innovations that would have been impossible to introduce in other cultures. Roman military physicians never lost sight of their goal, which was to reach as many wounded as quickly as possible and save as many as possible. They rejected anything that hindered that goal and continually searched for solutions.

The shortcoming of Roman medicine was that it never struck deep roots in Roman society. From beginning to end, it was always a product of the Roman military machine. And when that machine finally came to a halt and the empire collapsed, there were few resources within the society to preserve and transmit Roman medical skill to future generations. And much of what Rome had achieved in military medicine, as with so many other aspects of Roman civilization, was lost in the tide of barbarism that swept over Europe in the fifth century. The continuous upward trend of medical knowledge and civilization that had begun more than four millennia earlier in the Mesopotamian Valley came to a grinding halt. For the rest of the fifth century until the beginning of the Renaissance, the barbarian cultures of Europe produced nothing of medical value. The great legacy that was Rome vanished into a dark age that would take the West almost a thousand years from which to recover.

Notes

1. The date of 753 BCE is archaeologically too late to mark the first settlement of Rome and too early to mark the beginnings of genuine urbanization. It seems to have come into common use as a consequence of a squabble among ancient historians. See Michael Grant, *History of Rome* (New York: Charles Scribner, 1978), 10.

2. A good history of the early Italian military systems can be found in Connolly, *Greece and Rome at War*, 90–126.

3. G. R. Watson, *The Roman Soldier* (Ithaca, NY: Cornell University Press, 1969), 56.

4. On the Marian reforms, see Christopher Matthew, *On the Wings of Eagles: The Reforms of Gaius Marius and the Creation of Rome's First Professional Soldiers* (Newcastle upon Tyne, UK: Cambridge Scholars Publishing, 2010).

5. Garrison, *Introduction to the History of Medicine*, 105. Italians still have a cultural distrust of certain professions today. An old southern Italian proverb says that one ought never to trust doctors, lawyers, or priests, since they all make a living from other peoples' misery.

6. Garrison, *Notes on the History of Military Medicine*, 57.

7. Cicero notes that "raw recruits make shameful outcries over slight wounds, while the experienced seasoned soldier is pluckier and merely looks around for a surgeon to apply the dressing." Cicero, *Tusculan Disputation*, book 4, 16, 38.

8. Sir T. C. Allbutt, *Greek Medicine in Rome* (London: Macmillan, 1921), 21.

9. John Scarborough, "Roman Medicine and the Legions: A Reconsideration," *Medical History* 12, no. 3 (1968): 255. This is an excellent source for Roman military medical care before the establishment of the medical service under Augustus.

10. Scarborough quotes Polibius, book 2, 66.9, on this point. In modern military psychiatry, such behavior is evidence of "silent psychiatric casualties." After World War I, the British Army studied its manpower losses due to gas attacks. Its study revealed that almost 65 percent of those claiming injury from gas attacks either had suffered no such attack or, more frequently, had spread a small amount of mustard gas residue on their skin and reported to the medical tent. Similar indications of a desire to avoid combat include high rates of frostbite and hand injuries, known in the American army of World War II as M-1 thumb, prior to battle. See Gabriel, *No More Heroes*, chapter 3.

11. Scarborough, "Roman Medicine and the Legions," 256.

12. Ibid., 257.

13. Garrison, *Notes on the History of Military Medicine*, 52. After the battle of Gettysburg, more than 24,000 wounded from both sides were left behind to be cared for by a population of less than twenty-four hundred townspeople.

14. Livy notes this practice with regard to the Volscians (book 4, 39) and the Carthaginians (book 7, 8).

15. Livy, book 2, 17.

16. Tiberius, for example, provided doctors and litters at his own expense. Germanicus actually tended some of the wounded himself. Trajan paid for the medical care of the army out of his own pocket, and Aurelian made medical care a right for any wounded soldier.

17. H. H. Huxley, "Greek Doctor and Roman Patient," *Greece and Rome* 4, no. 2 (October 1957): 132–38. Pliny says of Archagathus that "soon he came to be feared by the Romans because of his cruel methods of treatment . . . because of his cruelty in cutting and burning."

18. Garrison, *Notes on the History of Military Medicine*, 60.

19. Majno, *Healing Hand*, 390.

20. This said, the earliest epigraphical evidence for the presence of doctors in the army is a votive tablet by Sextus Titius Alexander, *medicus* of the Fifth Praetorian Cohort, dedicated to "Asclepius and the health of his comrades."

21. Garrison, *Notes on the History of Military Medicine*, 62.

22. Vivian Nutton, "Medicine and the Roman Army: A Further Consideration," *Medical History* 13, no. 3 (1969): 266.

23. George Rosen, *A History of Public Health* (New York: MD Publications, 1958), 47.

24. Two of the most famous Roman physicians were military physicians—Cornelius Celsus, who gave us a manual of wound surgery, and Pedanius Dioscorides, who left us the most complete materia medica of the ancient world. Ackerknecht, *Short History of Medicine*, 72.

25. Garrison, *Notes on the History of Military Medicine*, 67.

26. Ibid.

27. For an excellent work on the surgeon in the Roman army, including his training, texts, instruments, and clinical skill, see Ralph Jackson, *The Surgeon and the Army* (Norman: University of Oklahoma Press, 1988).

28. Watson, *The Roman Soldier*, 39.

29. Orville Oughtred, "How the Romans Delivered Medical Care along Hadrian's Wall Fortifications," *Michigan Medicine* 79, no. 5 (February 1980): 59.

30. Jackson, *The Surgeon and the Army*, 105.

31. The similarities between Varro's theory of disease and the later germ theory put forward by Koch are striking. Varro notes that the cause of disease had the following characteristics: (1) the pathogen is animal, (2) it is alive, (3) it is too small to be seen, (4) it is airborne, (5) it enters the body, (6) it emanates from swamps, (7) it produces not one disease but many, and (8) these diseases are refractory. For more on Varro and his concept of disease, see Saul Jarcho, "Medical and Nonmedical Comments on Cato and Varro, with Historical Observations on the Concept of Infection," *Transactions and Studies of the College of Physicians of Philadelphia* 43, no. 4 (1976): 372–78.

32. Reginald Hargreaves, "The Long Road to Military Hygiene," *The Practitioner* 196 (March 1966): 439.

33. The Roman fort is described in detail in Roy Davies, *Service in the Roman Army* (New York: Columbia University Press, 1989), 211.

34. For a description of the Assyrian medical service see Adamson, "The Military Surgeon," 44–45.

35. See Scarborough, "Roman Medicine and the Legions"; Nutton, "Medicine and the Roman Army"; and Jackson, *The Surgeon and the Army*, on this point.

36. The Union Army trained its own physicians during the Civil War. Paradoxically, the South closed its medical schools without providing alternative training in the military, resulting in a critical shortage of trained medical personnel.

37. Davies, *Service in the Roman Army*, 214.

38. Ibid.

39. The term is derived from the little pouches or boxes (*capsa*) containing the bandages and dressings that the medics carried. It is the first instance that we know of where combat medics used standard-issue field kits.

40. Gabriel, "Trajan's Column," 43.

41. Richard A. Gabriel, "The Roman Military Medical Corps," *Military History*, January 2011, 39–44. One of the reasons that the wounded often died on the battlefield is that no one could find them to treat them. It often took days to locate a wounded soldier, during which time he often succumbed. Designating combat medics specifically to locate the wounded quickly and move them to the field hospital was a major advance in the treatment of the wounded.

42. Juliane C. Wilmanns, *Der Sanitätsdienst im Römischen Reich: Eine sozialgeschichtliche Studie zum römischen Militärsanitätswesen nebst einer Prosopographie des Sanitätspersonals* (Zurich: Medizin der Antike 2, 1995).

43. These same principles are used to guide the application of military psychiatry in the field. See Gabriel, *No More Heroes*, chapter 4.

44. Davies, *Service in the Roman Army*, 213–14.

45. Ibid.

46. Ibid.

47. Garrison, *Notes on the History of Military Medicine*, 65.

48. For example, the Roman hospital at Inchtuthil in England was constructed to handle a minimal casualty rate of 12.5 percent, or considerably more than the 2–5 percent that was usually planned for. See Nutton, "Medicine in the Roman Army," 263.

49. Davies, *Service in the Roman Army*, 220–21.

50. See Rudolf Schultz, "Die römische Legionen lazarette in Vetera und andersen Legionslagern" *Bonn Journal* 139 (1934): 54–63, for the complete analysis and archaeology of the Roman military hospital at Vetera, Germany.

51. Just how the Romans came to sterilize surgical instruments as a standard medical practice is unknown. On the one hand, it may have been an extension of the fastidious Roman concern for cleanliness. On the other hand, Galen recommended sterilization perhaps as a consequence of noticing some connection between cleanliness and the onset of infection.

52. Hippocrates had used special diets for convalescence extensively.

53. Davies, *Service in the Roman Army*, 219–29, for a detailed description of the Roman military hospital.

54. Ackerknecht, *Short History of Medicine*, 72–73.

55. Majno, *Healing Hand*, 374–81.

56. Ibid.

57. There is little doubt that army doctors used both Celsus's and Dioscorides's works as medical texts.

58. After the collapse of the empire and the barbarian invasions, the Catholic Church placed religious restrictions upon dissection for a time, leading once more to the decline of anatomical knowledge. Da Vinci, for example, had to conduct his dissections in secret and write his notes backward to prevent translation and avoid punishment at the hands of the religious and secular authorities.

59. Roman knowledge of the circulatory system was derived from the knowledge first produced by the Alexandrian school researchers.

60. Aldea and Shaw, "Evolution of the Surgical Management," 550.

61. Majno, *Healing Hand*, 387.

62. Salazar, *The Treatment of War Wounds*, 60–61.

63. Jackson, *The Surgeon and the Army*, 112.

64. Salazar, *Treatment of War Wounds*, 61.

65. Celsus's famous description of the ideal surgeon clearly makes the point. The surgeon, he says, "needs to be compassionate, but not to the extent that, moved by the latter's cries, he either hurries more than is required or cuts less than necessary, but he must do everything just as if no sympathy were aroused in him by the other's [the patient's] screams." Ibid., 64.

66. Roman surgical instruments were made of copper, brass, and iron. By the imperial period, Roman metallurgy had advanced to where instruments were made of fine surgical steel.

67. The instrument used for arrow extraction is mentioned by Celsus as being the "spoon of Diokles," suggesting that it was of Greek origin. Diodorus says that a physician named Critobulus of Cos used the instrument to extract the arrow that wounded Philip II of Macedonia at the siege of Methone in 354 BCE. Gabriel, *Philip II of Macedonia*, 13–14.

68. Hospital-acquired postsurgical infection remains a major problem in modern times. Physicians themselves are the primary source of infections by failing to

wash their hands before touching their patients, and that was the same cause of infection in hospitals at the turn of the last century.

69. Jackson, *The Surgeon and the Army*, 113.
70. Majno, *Healing Hand*, 400.
71. Ibid., 188.
72. Ibid., 369.
73. Jackson, *The Surgeon and the Army*, 126.
74. Ibid.

10

BARBARIANS AND BYZANTINES, 478–1453 CE

The period from the first through the second centuries CE was the high point in the development of military medicine in the ancient world. In its degree of medical knowledge and its ability to deliver medical care to the wounded soldier, Roman military medicine was not surpassed until modern times and in some aspects not until World War II. Chapters 10 and 11 examine military medicine from the third century to the fifteenth century, a period in which the medical arts retrogressed to Bronze Age times. The single exception to this decline was the Byzantine Empire (395–1453 CE), where military medicine continued to be practiced with clinical excellence. Even under the Byzantines, however, medical knowledge and practice were frozen as if in cold storage, until the West was ready to use them again during the Renaissance.

The third through fifteenth centuries were marked by near-total disintegration of Western culture. Most of the major social, political, economic, and military institutions that had taken the West more than a thousand years to develop were lost in a tide of barbarian invasions and religious intolerance of scientific thought. Medical knowledge and innovation came to a halt. The once-civilized Roman West plunged into a long dark night that was only briefly punctuated by flashes of scientific light that produced anything of lasting value. The disintegration and decentralization of all aspects of social life were the chief characteristics of this period. Clinical medicine was either destroyed or rigorously suppressed until little of value remained. The destruction of everyday technology—water systems and sewage, roads, education, food supplies, communications, and so on—was so complete that social technology was reduced to levels not seen in Europe for almost a thousand years. The degree of technological collapse can be compared to the state of affairs that might exist a hundred years after a nuclear attack on the current, sophisticated social orders of Europe.[1]

The confusion of this barbarian and Byzantine age presents a problem as to how to organize the analysis of military medicine in this period. Chapters 10 and 11 are arranged into four chronologies that are distinct in time and place; however, they are somewhat artificial in that they construct barriers that did not truly exist in the minds of those who lived during this time. Nonetheless, in order not to repeat the era's hopeless confusion in the analysis, some organizational schema is necessary.

The first period encompasses the third to the eighth centuries, when successive waves of barbarian invasion, settlement, and reinvasion destroyed the Roman Empire and its organizational structure in the West. This period is marked by the total eclipse of the Roman military medical system, accompanied by drastic changes in military forms, and its replacement by a primitive but widely used form of tribal military medicine. The second period focuses on the Byzantine Empire with its capital at Constantinople (395–1453 CE). Here, the medical knowledge of the West and the Roman military medical system were preserved for almost a thousand years after the collapse of the Roman military system in the West. While little in the way of medical innovations can be credited to the Byzantines, their preservation of the medical knowledge of the ancients and the spread of that knowledge to the Muslim Empire was vital to the renewed development of military medicine during the Renaissance. The third period addresses military medicine as practiced by the armies of Islam and the transmission of that knowledge to the West as a consequence of their cultural and military contacts with a degraded Europe. The character and value of Islamic medicine have been generally overstated, in further testimony to the low level to which medical knowledge and practice had fallen in the West. The last period of analysis addresses medicine in the Middle Ages, the period beginning with the Carolingian Empire of Charlemagne (800 CE) and the rise of feudalism and ending with the dawn of the Renaissance in the fourteenth century, when military medicine began to reemerge in the West.

The Barbarians

Writing in 1744 CE, Ferdinando Galliani noted that "empires being neither up nor down do not fall. They change their appearance."[2] The barbarian invasions of the Roman Empire for the first four centuries match this description precisely. Rome did not collapse as much as it metamorphosed into a decentralized state of quasi-Romanized Germanic fiefdoms, each ruled by a warlord supported by a private army. The Roman army always had to deal with the problem of hostile tribes on its boundaries. In Gaul, Spain, and Britain, Rome solved the problem through military conquest and the eventual Romanization of the tribal peoples in these areas. The problem on the German frontier, however, was different. Here the tribes were very large, were culturally warlike, offered nothing in terms of resources that could be obtained by conquest, and occupied an area of dense forest, rivers, and mountainous terrain that was difficult to control. The destruction of three Roman legions at the hands of the German tribal chieftain Arminius in 9 CE in the Teutoburg Forest effectively settled the problem of German conquest for the Romans.[3] Afterward, Roman military strategy in the region changed to the defensive and was marked by the creation of a system of in-depth fortifications constructed along the German frontier.[4]

The Roman defensive strategy succeeded in repelling the Germans' repeated attempts at penetration throughout the first and second centuries. It was not until 260 CE, when the Franks moved into Spain, the Alamanni pressed into the Alvergne country, and the Goths crossed the Danube River in large numbers, that the first significant incursions succeeded. The Roman army, long garrisoned along the imperial frontiers, had begun to decay. Many of the frontier posts had become large towns with substantial civilian contingents within them.[5] Training and discipline declined. By the second century, not more than 1 percent of the Roman army comprised native Italians, with the rest having been drawn from other nationalities of the empire socialized to Roman values and methods. By the middle of the third century, the Roman army could no longer meet the invasion threat. The German tribes broke through in great numbers and settled sizable tracts of imperial land.[6]

The Romans' response was to reorganize the army with militia troops (the *limitani*), garrison the local forts, and hold large horse-borne reserves at key rear garrisons that could rush to a point of penetration and throw the enemy back. By this time, though, most of the army comprised barbarian soldiers in the pay of Rome. As Roman reliance upon these barbarian military forces grew, the legions' organizational structure eroded until, by the fourth century, they were no longer formed along traditional Roman lines. Instead, they reflected barbarian weapons, tactics, values, and formations, and they were commanded by their own tribal chiefs. This arrangement continued until the fifth century when renewed waves of barbarian invasions crashed over Europe, effectively putting an end to the Roman military system.

The gradual barbarization of the legions had an enormous impact on Roman military organization.[7] The decline in the legion's administrative and support structure led to its replacement by barbarian military practices that precipitated a collapse of the legion's military medical structure. As early as the third century, the declining quality of the defensive outposts along the Rhine had turned the once-magnificent Roman military hospitals into little more than "rudimentary sick bays."[8] By 250 CE, the names of Roman military doctors who had occupied such a prominent place in the legion's official records and had appeared on scores of burial monuments all but disappeared, suggesting that the medical service was in serious decline.[9] By 325 CE, more evidence appeared that the Roman medical service was chronically short of medical personnel. While conducting a campaign along the Danube, the emperor Valentinian suffered a minor hemorrhage that required medical attention. The campaign records note that the emperor did not have a physician to attend him in the field because available medical personnel were in the camp fighting an outbreak of disease.[10]

By 350 CE, the Roman military medical system had almost disintegrated. The poor state of its military medical care is testified to by Ammianus Marcellinus's account of the battle between Julian and the Chionites. The chronicler notes that after the battle "each side looked after its wounded as best they could," depending on the number of *curantes* available.[11] The curantes to whom medical treatment was now entrusted were low-level attendants. The term for military medical doctor, *medicus,* had disappeared from the records almost a century earlier. Marcellinus's account would seem to indicate that the trained military physician was no longer a regular figure in the army. He also documents the depths to which the quality of Roman military field medicine had fallen when he says that many of the wounded bled to death because no one present knew how to stop the bleeding.[12] Given that two of the major advances of the old Roman military medical service were its abilities to use the tourniquet and to suture arteries, Marcellinus certainly indicates a decline in Roman field medicine. Moreover, he notes that many of the wounded could not have the arrows and lances withdrawn from their bodies and died where they fell.[13] The ability of the old Roman medical service to extract arrows and other missiles had been a high art, and its absence in this account further suggests the low point to which field medicine had fallen. The evidence indicates that by 350 CE the Roman medical service no longer existed in any organized form.

At the Battle of Chalôns (451 CE) a century later, the Roman medical service had completely disappeared. Records of the battle between Atilla and a coalition of western Frank and Gallic tribes allied with Rome demonstrate that the "Roman" armies of the West no longer had any medical support. Tim Newark notes in his account of the battle's aftermath that the men had no ability to extract arrows and other projectiles, that shock and bleeding took a heavy toll, and that infection and putrefaction were common.[14] Alas, the old Roman military medical corps had excelled precisely in treating these conditions.

With the death of the Roman military medical service, no one was left in the West to preserve the knowledge and skills of empirical medicine. The Roman civilian medical establishment was ill equipped for the task. Medicine had neither been held in high esteem nor struck deep roots in Roman society. Medical education was concentrated in civilian societies or "colleges" that became formalized with the establishment of the Medicorum schola under Vespasian (70–79 CE).[15] Roman civilian medicine was free from the press of treating battle wounds and tended to focus on the general practice of medicine rather than on battle surgery.[16] It is unlikely that Roman civilian doctors ever attained the same degree of surgical skill that their military counterparts developed. Moreover, Roman civilian medicine reflected a high level of traditional folk medicine and other nonempirical aspects of medical practice. The temples of Asculepias and other pagan temple practitioners competed for the physician's business until Constantine closed them in 335 CE. By that time, however, the practice of medicine was already falling into the hands of Christian monks. While the secular medical establishment continued to exist, it was never in a position to be the caretaker of the highly developed surgical knowledge and skill that had been the military physician's domain. Roman clinical medicine had been a creation of the legions, and when the legions collapsed, the practice of effective military medicine died with them.

The armies of the West became thoroughly barbarized in all respects, and it should come as no surprise that these armies practiced a form of military medicine that was rooted in their tribal customs. The cultural level of military forces, along with the general societies of the West, plunged back into one reminiscent of the Bronze Age, with the result that the practice of military medicine available to the Western barbarized armies was even less effective than the primitive, proto-empirical medicine that the ancient Sumerians had practiced.

The German "medical system" serves as an interesting example. As a tribal culture, the Germanics were pagans with a strong belief in demons and in the curative powers of magicians and shamans.[17] As many of these practitioners were women, there grew in Germanic lore the tradition of *wilde Weiber* (wild women), who could cure battle wounds by chanting incantations, preparing poultices, and sucking the poison from wounds. Germanic medical practitioners believed in the curative properties of certain magical herbs, parts of animals, and votive foods.[18] As tribal armies, Germanic armies were accompanied by large contingents of women, family members, and other camp followers who treated the wounded. This practice continued to at least the eighth century and perhaps beyond.[19]

The role of women in the medical care system of the tribal armies raises an interesting point. Women in the medieval period serving as nurses, especially in the founding of convent orders to treat the sick, is often attributed to the influence of the Catholic Church, which, because of its veneration of Mary as the mother of God, provided women a place in the social order that they had previously lacked. While there is some truth to this assertion, it may equally have been that the central presence of women as caregivers in the barbarian armies from time immemorial was the cultural force that allowed women to play an important role in medical caregiving in the Middle Ages.[20]

It is important to emphasize that the quality of medical care provided to the barbarian armies of this period was almost useless in a clinical sense. Unlike the Greeks, who used a semi-empirical pharmacology in wound treatment, the Germans' use of various herbs and poultices was essentially an exercise in magic. Moreover, the wilde Weiber could do little for bleeding or shock, and their habit of stuffing a wound with all kinds of materials to effect a cure probably made death by infection a certainty.[21] With the demise of the Roman military medical system, these tribal medical practices eventually had no competitors, as even the Roman civilian medical system collapsed and disappeared. Meanwhile, the terrible destruction and constant warfare that characterized this period led to an ever more important role for the papacy in the lives of the converted Christian warriors, tribes, and feudal realms. The tenor of the times coupled with the newness of the still-developing Christian religion plunged medicine into fear and ignorance. Since only the clergy had the time or inclination to practice medicine, medical practice between the fifth and ninth centuries fell almost entirely into the hands of the newly founded monastic orders.

Although the quality of wound treatment provided to the soldiers of this period was low, it is noteworthy that at least some efforts were made to treat the wounded. The *idea* of military medicine did not die with the loss of medical knowledge. Evidence from the fourth century in the Crimea shows that Scythian chiefs made attempts to bandage wounds, and the Norse sagas reference the use of herbs and cauterization for battle wounds.[22] A passage in the *Nibelungenlied* notes that the king of Burgundy looked after the care and transportation of his wounded vassals, although no provisions are mentioned for the common soldier.[23] Some medical attendants were in evidence as professional leechers who bled the soldiers and were paid "silver and bright gold" for their efforts.[24]

Medical knowledge had declined to desperate states, and clinical practice fell into the hands of monastics, some of whose orders were founded to treat illness and disease. Medicine of this time faced a difficult road, and the church's insistence that faith, prayers, and fasting were better remedies than those of powerless physicians did little to foster sound medical practice. The practice of medicine by clerics and monks led to a number of fatal abuses that drove the reputation of medicine and especially surgery even lower, until the practice of surgery almost died out altogether.[25] To curtail what had become barbarous and mostly fatal medical practices, the Catholic Church issued a number of decrees that, although unintended, damaged the reputation of medicine even further. In their various codes of law (Visogothic Code, fifth–ninth centuries), the civic authorities also imposed stiff penalties, including execution, upon physicians who caused their patients' deaths. The result was that surgery, formerly the most useful aspect of military medical practice, fell into such disrepute that it was left mostly to barbers (*barbitonsores*) who had received their training by bleeding and shaving monks.[26]

As surgery and medicine fell increasingly into disrepute, the hospital movement began to emerge.[27] As early as 361 CE, the church and even public authorities began to establish hospitals to treat the sick, the wars' casualties, and those suffering from illnesses caused by a decline in diet and epidemics provoked by the collapse of the Roman system of public hygiene.[28] For the most part, however, these hospitals did not provide any actual medical treatment, and few doctors were in evidence. The sick were given food and prayers, usually until they died.[29] Not until the fourteenth century did hospitals actually offer some medical care and provide primitive mercury ointment treatments to combat the endemic syphilis of the population. By the year 1000 CE, the church hospitals began to decline because of a loss of revenue. They turned the task of ministering to the sick largely over to monastic orders as their obligation of charity.

With regard to the treatment of battle wounds, the clinical Greco-Roman medical tradition that Roman military physicians had so carefully fashioned was virtually lost to the practitioners of the day. What little work of the ancients that the monastic copiers of the period had preserved was almost useless. The translation movement did not get under way until the fourth century, and most of the books remained locked up in monastic libraries, preserved as objects of art and veneration, where they could not be read or disseminated. It required the invention of the printing press in the fifteenth century before this storehouse of medical knowledge could be dispersed sufficiently to form the basis of medical practice and education once again. Additionally, much of what the monastic translators had preserved was carefully scrutinized for elements of medical practice that were deemed contrary to the Christian faith. Those elements the church considered dangerous to the faith were excluded or altered to reflect current religious views. The result was that only a limited amount of accurate clinical information was transmitted to future generations.

Two medical procedures of primary importance in treating battle casualties, the art of ligature to stop blood loss and the prevention of infection, were completely lost during this period. The use of the tourniquet disappeared entirely until Ambroise Paré reintroduced it in the sixteenth century. Of even greater clinical importance, however, was an incorrect view of wound infection that probably killed more soldiers than shock and bleeding. Galen's works provided the one common medical text for educating physicians during this period, but unfortunately, much of what he had to say about anatomy was incorrect.[30] With regard to treating infection, however, Galen had soundly rejected the idea that infection was a natural part of the healing process.[31] Regrettably, the translation of Galen's works that strongly influenced medical practice during the Middle Ages was so inaccurate that instead Galen became the primary source that practitioners quoted on the need to ensure infection as a part of the natural wound-healing process. Although Roman military physicians had been masters at preventing infection of battle wounds, the advocates of necessary suppuration gained prominence in the Middle Ages with predictably disastrous results. It became standard medical practice to use all sorts of foul mixtures to pack open wounds in the hope that it would provoke *pus bonun et laudible*, which, of course, it did with devastating consequences. After the Renaissance, the deliberate stimulation of infection died out, but the idea that infection was a natural part of the healing process continued until Lister introduced the concept of antisepsis in the 1860s. The inability to stem bleeding and the deliberate provocation of infection combined to make the practice of military medicine far more dangerous than providing no treatment at all.

The persistence of Galen's influence also caused problems for hemostasis and some aspects of diagnosis. Galen believed that the blood ebbed and flowed in the arteries and veins; that is, the vessels were bidirectional channels in which blood flowed in both directions within the same conduit. Galen further maintained that the blood flowed from one side of the heart to the other through holes in the septum. For centuries, scientists deluded themselves that they had in fact seen such holes in order not to contradict Galen, even though no such holes existed. It was not until the mid-sixteenth century that Andreas van Wesel published a work challenging Galen's claim. Forty years later Girolamo Fabrizio in Padua discovered the valves in the veins that made bidirectional blood flow impossible. William Harvey was a doctoral student of Fabrizio's, and in 1628 Harvey published his famous *Exercitatio Anatomica de Motu Cordis et Sanguinis in Animalibus* in which he established the modern theory of circulation of the blood.[32]

Some idea of how far medical practice had fallen into mysticism can be gained by noting that the practice of exorcism as a cure for illness thrived during this period. In many ways, the church's emphasis on demons as a cause of illness resembled the practice of religious medicine in Babylon more than a thousand years earlier. The Babylonian emphasis on demons had been transmitted to the West through a number of Jewish religious sects during the Babylonian captivity. Although the Hebraic priesthood rejected such ideas and attempted to stamp out the practice, a strong belief in demons as causes of disease and illness survived in the Essene sect, with which, it is generally held, Christ was associated. The Babylonian emphasis on demons was thus transmitted directly to the Christian religion and, exacerbated as it was by the terrible political and social conditions of the early Middle Ages, reemerged in full bloom in the medical practices of the period.

Paintings of the period show monks arranged in a magic circle around a clerical physician performing an exorcism over a patient, who is often portrayed with a demon emerging from his or her mouth. It was also common practice to produce lists of diseases and the corresponding names of the specific demons responsible for causing each disease. Placed next to the list of diseases and demons was a list of saints whose magical powers could be beseeched by prayer to cure the illness. Under these conditions, medical science decayed remarkably.

The period in the West from the fourth century to the tenth century CE was a time when medical knowledge and the medical arts, especially surgery, sank to levels that had not been seen in the ancient world since before the Greek era. Indeed, in numerous instances the medical arts of Sumer and Egypt were considerably more clinically effective than was medicine in the Middle Ages. The efficient Roman military medical system had ceased to exist in all its important respects and had been replaced by a tribal medicine strongly influenced by superstition and magic. This tribal military medicine had nothing to recommend it in terms of clinical effectiveness and was only slightly more useful in providing some organizational means to provide medical care to the wounded. The introduction of a number of medical doctrines, the most important of which was the idea of natural infection, weighed heavily upon military medical practice until modern times. For all practical purposes, military medicine had ceased to exist in the armies of the West.

The Byzantine Empire

The centuries of invasion, civil war, and general decay took their fatal toll on the Roman Empire of the West. From the fourth century onward, the legacy of Rome was gradually transferred to its eastern capital, Constantinople, where Roman emperors attempted to stem the tide of barbarism and preserve the essence of Roman culture. By 650 CE, however, the empire of the East was forced to accept the loss of the western provinces and was confronted with numerous military threats from Islamic invaders. These threats occupied the empire's attention for the next eight hundred years. It is testimony to Byzantine greatness and skill that the empire survived and prospered for more than a millennium after the collapse of Rome until suffering its final defeat at the hand of Ottoman armies in 1453 CE. While the western Roman empire had lasted five hundred years, the eastern empire (395–1453 CE) had lasted for more than a thousand.

The imposition of Roman administrative machinery upon the Byzantine population in the early years kept the traditions of Roman military science and law intact and preserved Roman culture and achievement for more than a millennium until, as Allbutt noted, "Western Europe was once again fit to take care of them."[33] Byzantium suffered no period of general degradation as Europe did in the Middle Ages, and it remained the most refined and developed culture in the world until the end.

Vital to Byzantine survival was the maintenance of its military capability, which "was, in its day, the most efficient military body in the world."[34] Despite many evolutionary changes in its details, the Byzantine military machine remained thoroughly Roman in its organization and values, and it continued to produce excellent soldiers and commanders long after the legions had disappeared in the West. The basic administrative and tactical unit of the Byzantine army for both cavalry and infantry was the *numerus* (military unit), comprised of 300–400 men. Comparable to a combat battalion, each numerus was commanded by the Western equivalent of a colonel. A *turma* (division) comprised five to eight battalions commanded by a general. Two or three turmae could be combined into a corps under a *strategos* (senior general). The empire was geographically organized into *themes* (administrative provinces), each of which had a military commander responsible for its security with deliberately unclear lines between civil and military administration so as to give priority to military defense. For more than four centuries, the Byzantine army numbered approximately 150,000 men, who were almost evenly divided between infantry and cavalry forces.[35]

Military manpower was sustained through universal conscription. Recruiting and stationing military forces within each theme allowed commanders to enlist the best manpower. The army attracted the finest families for its soldiers and avoided the fatal mistake of the western empire, which had relied heavily on barbarian soldiers while the best Roman citizens served not at all. Moreover, whereas Rome had relied heavily on infantry until too late, the Byzantines adjusted to the new forms of mobile, mounted warfare and developed an excellent heavy cavalry of their own.[36] Byzantine military commanders were quick to adopt their enemies' weapons and tactics when appropriate. As the infantry legion had symbolized the might of Rome, the *cataphracti* (mounted, armored horsemen) came to symbolize the military might of Byzantium.

The organization and infrastructure of the Byzantine army was every bit as well organized and efficient as it had been under the old Roman legions. The army had organic supply and logistics trains made up of carts and pack animals to give it mobility; excellent siege craft capabilities, including the full range of Roman artillery and siege craft specialists; a fully articulated staff organization that was professionally trained in military academies; and a powerful navy to support ground operations. In Byzantium, the Romans' genius for military organization was preserved intact in almost all its earlier aspects.

Among the important surviving staff functions was the military medical service. Unlike Rome, where civilian medicine had not struck deep roots and was easily replaced by tribal and clerical medicine, clinical medicine reached high art among the Byzantine civilian medical establishment. It continued to use the medical texts of the Greeks and Romans, including the all-important military medical manuals, until the end of the empire. Indeed, civilization owes more to Byzantium's compilers and translators for treasuring and transmitting these medical texts to the modern world than it does to the efforts of the Western Christian monks who are often given credit for salvaging them from the barbarian invasions. Contrary to what occurred in the West under the impact of tribalism and religious superstition, the practice of medicine did not decline, and the Byzantine civil service constructed and operated a highly organized system of public health administration and public hospitals.[37] It was in Byzantium that the four-thousand-year-old tradition of clinical pragmatism was preserved for future generations.

Emperor Mauritius (582–602 CE) officially introduced the military medical corps into Byzantine military formations, and they represented more of a revised version of the old legion's medical service than the introduction of something entirely new. The decentralization of military formations organized by theme and the mobility required to successfully conduct large cavalry operations increased the need for more medical personnel than were required in the old, less mobile infantry legions. With a state-run medical service and medical schools helping the civilian populace, the Byzantines also had a much larger pool of trained physicians and other medical personnel from which to draw military medical assets. The resulting system could place more medical personnel in the service of the soldier in small units.

Under the Byzantines, each horse or cavalry battalion had its own medical detachment of two physicians—a general practitioner and a specialist in surgery. The medical staff was augmented by eight to eighteen medical orderlies who served as combat medics and stretcher bearers.[38] Thus, the Byzantine army continued to institute the principle of immediacy of treatment, first seen in the legions' use of combat medics. The Byzantine practice of constructing a fortified camp each evening while on the march also included a field hospital positioned near the battle lines to receive and treat casualties.

The *deputati* (medical orderlies) were unarmed, enjoyed noncombatant status, and served in numerous different roles depending upon need. Their primary function was to serve as combat medics. They generally positioned themselves two hundred to three hundred yards back from the fighting and remained ready to rush forward and bring the severely wounded to the rear for medical treatment. In cavalry units, and apparently in some infantry units as well, the deputati were provided with horses and special saddles with two ladder straps on the left side that could be used to carry the wounded to safety.[39] This arrangement gave the medical personnel a degree of mobility on the battlefield that was only duplicated with the introduction of motorized vehicles in modern times. Combat medics also carried bandages and water flasks as standard equipment and administered first aid to the wounded until a physician could be found.

In an army composed of the state's best citizens, who were used to excellent and easily available medical care in civilian life, the importance of military medical care to the army's morale and combat ability is repeatedly noted in the military commentaries of the Byzantines.[40] As incentives to perform under fire, medical personnel were given a financial bonus in gold for every wounded soldier they rescued from the fray and brought to the medical tent. These orderlies were also given a share of any booty that resulted from the battle.[41]

The level of public hygiene in Byzantium was certainly as good as it had been in Rome and in many respects better. Byzantines bathed at least once a day, and some elements of the population did as often as a three times a day. As a matter of course, then, military field hygiene was excellent, and a medical hygiene corps maintained many of the standard Roman practices. The Byzantine medical system of the state and church also provided for soldiers who had been severely wounded and invalided from service. The first tentative evidence of a system of long-term medical care for soldiers (the forerunners of the modern veterans' hospitals) is found in the claim that Constantine (306–337 CE) founded the first veterans' hospital. Justin II (565–578 CE) founded a hospital for crippled soldiers, and Alexis I Comnenus (1081–1118 CE) established a hospital for soldiers with long-term medical conditions.[42] These long-term care hospitals were a major advance in military medicine over Alexander's practice of providing a pension to the disabled and the Roman practice of establishing special colonies of wounded veterans and freeing them from certain taxes. For the first time in history, men disabled by war could look forward to an acceptable level of medical care for the rest of their lives. It was quite different from the eighteenth-century practices of the English army, which bestowed upon wounded soldiers discharged from service only a single benefit, the right to priority in obtaining beggar's licenses.

The quality of medical care under the Byzantine military medical system was every bit as good as it had been under the Romans but perhaps not much better.[43] While established medical science was preserved intact—similar to the monks in the West, the Byzantines were great compilers of medical texts—there does not appear to have been much in the way of medical innovation. The sixth book of Paul of Aegina (625–690 CE), the most famous and important Byzantine compiler, provided the definitive work on military surgery of the period and remained the standard source until the twelfth century.[44] While the compilations of Greek and Roman surgical procedures were excellent, the work offered nothing new. Its importance lay in the fact that it was passed directly to the Muslims in undiluted form, where it served as the basic medical text for later Muslim physicians.

If the advancement of medical knowledge and treatment came to a halt under the Byzantines, at least the clinical aspects of military medicine remained intact and highly empirical. Moreover, the medicine available to the soldier did not decline, as had happened in the West. The doctrine of laudible pus and deliberately provoked infection did not take serious hold in Byzantium, and battle surgery remained at a relatively high level. The level of military medicine was as effective as it had been under the old legions and perhaps even somewhat better given the greater number of medical assets available to smaller combat units.

Beyond military medicine, the world owes a great debt to the Byzantines for their roles as caretakers of the rich cultural and medical tradition of the West for more than a thousand years while the West was enduring its long, dark night following the collapse of Rome. History arranged for the Byzantines to become the major transmitters of this cultural heritage to the West and to act as an important influence on the development of Muslim medicine. The road was a twisting one, leading first to the Muslims and then back to the West. When Muslim medical texts reached the West in the eleventh and twelfth centuries, scholars were amazed at how advanced Muslim medical knowledge was. Had they not lost their own history, these Western scholars would have known that most Muslim medicine was nothing more than the old Greek and Roman clinical medicine practices that had been carefully preserved by the Byzantines, passed to the Muslim conquerors, and retransmitted to the West.[45]

The tale of the survival of Roman and Greek medicine begins with the fact that the Byzantines were great compilers of information, perhaps as befits history's caretakers. In 428 CE, an Assyrian-educated priest named Nestorius became the archbishop of Constantinople and immediately engaged the hierarchy of the church in a debate over the nature of Christ. In 431 CE, Nestorius and his followers were excommunicated for heresy and driven from Constantinople to settle in Edessa in Upper Mesopotamia. For almost thirty years, the Nestorian monks compiled and translated the major medical texts of the Greeks and Romans. In 489 CE, Emperor Zeno expelled them from the empire, and the Nestorian monks, thanks to the tolerance of the Persian king, settled in the town of Jundi-Shapur, bringing with them their valuable collection of Syriac translations of ancient Greek and Roman medical and scientific works.[46]

At Jundi-Shapur, the Nestorians also established a great university attached to a large teaching hospital. Its geographical setting allowed the university to become a unique meeting point of Persian, Greek, Alexandrian, Roman, Jewish, Hindu, and Chinese cultures. It was the greatest and most diverse university of its day and, under the tolerance of the Persian king, became the central storehouse for the world's medical knowledge, all of it carefully written down and preserved by the Nestorian monks. The university comprised three major schools: the School of Theology, Philosophy, and Metaphysics; the Institute of Translation, where masters presided over teams of translators fluent in all the major languages; and the teaching hospital, where students and physicians practiced medicine and did research.[47] This *bimaristan* (hospital) became the model used for all the great hospitals that the Muslims subsequently established in Baghdad, Damascus, and Cairo.

By 642 CE, the victorious Muslim armies had subdued all of Persia. The largely illiterate Arabs were impressed by the monks' work and recognized the value of the university.[48] Certainly they recognized the value of the hospital and, having no hospitals of their own, adopted the provision of free hospitals to the poor as fulfilling the Quranic obligation to treat the less fortunate. In the eighth century, the Omayyads sponsored the earliest known translations of Greek and Roman medical works from Syriac into Arabic.[49] At about the same time, the Muslim hospital movement began in earnest. In 756 CE, Al-Mansur, the founder of Baghdad, undertook a major effort to translate the entire collection of Jundi-Shapur into Arabic. As detailed in chapter 11, these texts formed the basis of Muslim medicine. Meanwhile, the store of Greek and Roman medical knowledge had been significantly augmented by additional knowledge and techniques drawn from Hindu and Chinese medicine. As the result of Muslim contacts with the West, this treasure trove of medical knowledge and clinical practices finally found its way back to Europe.

Notes

1. Some idea of how much technology declined following the collapse of the Roman Empire is found in Gabriel, *Culture of War,* chapter 8.

2. Galini is quoted in Tim Newark, *The Barbarians: Warriors and Wars of the Dark Ages* (London: Blanford Press, 1985), 51.

3. The seriousness with which the Romans regarded the German threat is evident in the policy of stationing almost a third of the total legionary force along the German frontier.

4. For an analysis of the strategic consequences of the Roman defeat at the Teutoburg Forest, see Gabriel, *Empires at War*, 2:532–42.

5. Mainz and Cologne are two examples.

6. The best work on how the Romans accommodated the press of German settlers during the empire is still Walter Goffart, *Barbarians and Romans, A.D. 418–584: Techniques of Accommodation* (Princeton, NJ: Princeton University Press, 1980).

7. Ibid., 216.

8. Laffont, *Ancient Art of Warfare*, 1:134.

9. Garrison, *Notes on the History of Military Medicine*, 78.

10. Ibid., 79.

11. "Each side looked after its wounded as best it could and according to the number of *curantes*; some, severely wounded, and bleeding to death, reluctantly breathed their last; others, transfixed by spears and fallen to the ground, were cast aside, as if corpses; others had so many wounds that it was forbidden to do anything for them, that these suffering ones should not be further tormented by useless manhandling; many, on account of the uncertain issue in the withdrawal of weapons from wounds, suffered agony worse than death." Ammianus Marcellinus, *Rerum Gestarum,* book XIX, 215.

12. Ibid.

13. Ibid.

14. Newark, *The Barbarians*, 26.

15. George Podgorny, "Islamic-Persian Medical Education," *North Carolina Medical Journal* 27, no. 3 (March 1966): 136.

16. Rosen, *History of Public Health*, 47. By the second century CE, Roman authorities had established a public medical service. These public health physicians were known as *archiatri* and were appointed to various towns and districts. In 160 CE, Antonius Pius regulated the assignment of public health officials, decreeing that large cities were to have ten officials, medium cities seven, and small towns no more than five. Their principal duty was to provide medical care to the poor. It is unlikely, however, that the archiatri had received a full medical education. More likely, they were medical orderlies of some sort, perhaps similar to modern-day nurses and medics.

17. For the role of magic in Germanic tribal culture, see Valerie I. J. Flint, *The Rise of Magic in Early Medieval Europe* (Oxford, UK: Clarendon Press, 1991).

18. One of these sacred curative foods was a thin, hard bread in the shape of a straight rod. After the Germans were converted to Christianity, the shape of this straight rod changed to three circles joined at the center, to reflect the Trinity. This new shape still exists today in the form of the pretzel.

19. Garrison, *Introduction to the History of Medicine*, 170–71.

20. In fact, the status of women under Greek and Roman law was much higher and included more rights, including property rights, than was the case under Christianity during the Middle Ages. What the church accomplished during this period was to formalize the position of women as it existed in the Germanic tribal societies, where they were valued as child bearers and nurses of men but had no significant legal or property rights.

21. Richard D. Forrest, "Development of Wound Therapy from the Dark Ages to the Present," *Journal of the Royal Society of Medicine* 75 (April 1982): 268–69. The practice of stuffing the wound with foul substances had its origins in Babylonian medicine, where it was believed that demons possessed the sick. The idea was to make the patient's body so repulsive that the demon would leave and take the illness with it. Given the church's belief in demons as causes of illness during this period and the tribal nature of Germanic medicine, it is not surprising that this practice gained wide currency in Europe during the Middle Ages.

22. Garrison, *Introduction to the History of Medicine*, 177.

23. Ibid.

24. Ibid.

25. Once the practice of medicine fell into the hands of monastics, the church became concerned about a number of abuses, including offenses against modesty, causing the death of patients, greed, and diverting the attention of the doctor-monks from the religious life. The practice of surgery had become so barbarous and dangerous that a number of feudal rulers enacted strict punishment codes for malpractice. Some of these punishments made the Hammurabi Code seem mild by comparison.

26. Many "surgeons" began as barbers shaving monk's tonsures and beards. So dangerous had surgery become that at the Council of Tours (1163 CE), the church issued the edict *Ecclesia Abhorret a Singuine* (the church does not shed blood), a doctrine that achieved the final separation between surgery and general medicine, thus formalizing a distinction that lasted another six hundred years. The immediate consequence was to drive the practice of surgery almost out of existence as a branch of medicine.

27. The initial stimulus for these hospitals came from the spread of endemic leprosy. Gregory of Tours established the first leprosarium in 560 CE. These institutions

were built more as isolation compounds, based on the ancient Hebraic idea of quarantine and isolation, than as hospitals intent on rendering medical treatment in any true sense.

28. The spread of epidemics during this period can be attributed to a number of factors, including the movement of rural populations and their animals into fortified towns where they continued many of their unhygienic practices. Students and soldiers wandering from one town to another often carried disease with them. The habit of depositing feces in any convenient spot and burying the dead in cemeteries within the city walls also contributed to the spread of disease.

29. This focus on prayer gave rise to a belief in the curative powers of relics, which became big business. The death of a powerful nobleman was often quickly followed by a declaration of his sainthood. It led to the practice of disinterring the body, boiling it down to its skeleton, and selling off the bones as relics. Neighboring monasteries sometimes fought armed clashes over the possession of relics.

30. Galen was more interested in internal medicine than in surgery, and his observations were drawn from the dissection of Barbary apes. Galen is important in ancient medicine because he was the first genuine clinical, medical, experimental scientist.

31. Galen's position on this issue is clear: "Those who believe that inflammation necessarily follows a wound show great ignorance." Majno, *Healing Hand*, 400.

32. See G. Whitteridge's translation of William Harvey's work of the same title (London: Blackwell Scientific Publications, 1976).

33. T. C. Allbutt, *Science and Medical Thought* (London: C. J. Clay and Sons, 1901), 65.

34. Charles Oman, *A History of the Art of War in the Middle Ages* (London: Methuen, 1898), book 3, chapter 1.

35. For a description of the Byzantine military system, see Dupuy and Dupuy, *Encyclopedia of Military History,* 215–16; and Gabriel, *Empires at War*, 3:987–1027. The military skill of the Byzantines is clearly displayed in a number of military treatises that have come down to us. One of the best English translations (along with the Greek passages) is George T. Dennis, *Three Byzantine Military Treatises* (Washington, DC: Dumbarton Oaks Press, Research Library and Collection, 1985).

36. The Byzantines did make use of various barbarian peoples as auxiliary units, but the excellent Byzantine intelligence service carefully watched them.

37. Timothy S. Miller, "Byzantine Hospitals," *Dumbarton Oaks Papers*, Symposium on Byzantine Medicine 38 (1984): 53–63. See also by the same author, *The Birth of the Hospital in the Byzantine Empire* (Baltimore: Johns Hopkins University Press, 1985).

38. Garrison, *Notes on the History of Military Medicine*, 79.

39. Ibid.

40. A description of the church-state hospital system in Byzantium is found in Tamara Talbot Rice, *Everyday Life in Byzantium* (New York: Putnam, 1967), 71–74.

41. Dupuy and Dupuy, *Encyclopedia of Military History*, 220.

42. Garrison, *Notes on the History of Military Medicine*, 81.

43. An understanding of the quality of Byzantine medicine, surgery, and pharmacology can be gained from exploring Owsei Temkin, "Byzantine Medicine: Tradition and Empiricism," *Dumbarton Oaks Papers* 16 (1962): 95–115. Also see the following articles, all produced at the Dumbarton Oaks Symposium on Byzantine Medicine in 1984: John Scarborough, "Early Byzantine Pharmacology," 213–32; Jerry Stannard, "Aspects of Byzantine Materia Medica," 205–11; Gerhard Baader, "Early Medieval Latin Adaptations of Byzantine Medicine in Western Europe," 251–59; John Duffy, "Byzantine Medicine in the Sixth and Seventh Centuries: Aspects of Teaching and Practice," 21–27; and Lawrence J. Bliquez, "Two Lists of Greek Surgical Instruments and the State of Surgery in Byzantine Times," 187–204.

44. Ibid.

45. De Lacey O'Leary, *How Greek Science Passed to the Arabs* (London: Routledge and K. Paul, 1949).

46. Podgorny, "Islamic-Persian Medical Education," 136–38.

47. Ibid., 138.

48. I have made a distinction here between Arabs and Muslims. In the early days of the Islamic conquests, the armies were Arab armies coming from Arabia and made up mostly of ethnic Arabian peoples. As conversions to Islam grew, the armies gradually incorporated the peoples of other lands who had become Muslims by accepting the Islamic faith. Thus, the armies that conquered Constantinople were Muslim in their faith but Turkic in their ethnicity.

49. Podgorny, "Islamic-Persian Medical Education," 139.

11

ISLAM AND THE MIDDLE AGES, 600–1453 CE

As the Byzantine Empire reached the peak of its cultural and military power in the seventh century, a power was stirring deep within the deserts of Arabia that would change the face of the world forever. To the Byzantines, the desert tracts of Arabia offered little rewards for conquest. Like their Persian contemporaries, the eastern Romans made no effort to control the area. Arabia's only wealth was found in a few merchant towns such as Mecca and Medina that sat astride the trade routes in the south. Into this world of Arab merchants and pastoral herdsmen a man destined to change the face of the world was born. His name was Mohammed, the founder of the religion of Islam.

Islam

Beginning with a small band of zealot followers who started raiding the caravan routes, Mohammed forged the beginnings of an Arab army that within a hundred years controlled all the territory from the Indus to the Atlantic along the North African littoral through Spain and to the border of southern France. Propelled by the belief that dying in war for the faith, or the jihad, gained one paradise in the next life, the armies of Islam gathered converts by the thousands wherever they marched.[1] By 732 CE, a century after Mohammed's death, the armies of Islam had destroyed the Persian Sassanid Empire, rolled back Byzantine power in the east to the Turkish border, incorporated all of Spain into the imperial realm, and narrowly missed overrunning France.[2]

No one could have foreseen this staggering degree of military success. Before Mohammed, Arab armies were hardly armies at all. The early followers of Mohammed were desert tribes and clans called to the banner of the faith, although they did not fight in organized formations. The idea of individual glory and faith drove warriors to feats of great bravery but at the same time made it impossible to organize as fighting units.[3] For more than a century, Arab soldiers fought with primitive weapons—the personal sword, dagger, and lance—and did not wear any defensive armor or helmets. These forces had no staff organization, no siege craft capabilities, and no logistics trains. Tactics were almost nonexistent as these armies relied upon small *razzias* (hit-and-run raids) and ambushes as their primary tactical maneuvers. Mobility was limited as most of the army moved on foot and fought as infantry, accompanied by small contingents of horse cavalry.[4] The size of these early armies was remarkably small. The force that attacked and subdued Egypt (640–642 CE) numbered no more than four thousand men.

Arab military development was influenced by experience and contact with other military cultures, most particularly the wars with the Byzantines and the Persians. In 635, Arab chieftain Khalid Ibn al-Walid, called the Sword of Allah, reorganized the Arab armies along Byzantine lines and created small combat units to replace the tribal levies. Whereas the tribes had deployed in lines only three men deep, al-Walid created dense infantry formations after the Byzantine pattern. These new formations were organized into archer, infantry, and lance cavalry units and put under the command of proven combat leaders who replaced the tribal and clan chiefs. He created the first Arab quartermaster corps and organized women to carry knives and short swords to strip and dispatch the enemy wounded.[5]

The early Arab armies relied upon camels for transport and cavalry. When the wars with the Persians brought the Arabs into contact with the horse, the warriors of Allah were quick to grasp the animal's importance as a military asset.[6] Since Arab horses were brought into regular contact with camels, the smell of the camel had no effect on them, whereas the Arabs' camel cavalry often spooked their enemies' horses and weakened their charge.

The Arab Empire reached its geographic zenith with its defeat by Charles Martel at the Battle of Poitiers in 732. Its expansionist phase over, the empire settled down to seven centuries of relative tranquility, punctuated by violent caliphate rebellions and border wars. The empire's defensive cast during this period was marked by its decentralization into a number of rival caliphates and the construction of *ribats* (military towns) that contained special units of religious warriors to protect the empire and the faith.[7] At the same time, however, Arab armies adopted more and more Persian and Byzantine military equipment and practices. By the tenth century, the chronicler al-Tabari recorded that Arab warriors carried the following equipment: mail armor, breastplate, helmet, leg and arm guards, complete horse armor, small shield, lance, sword, mace, battle ax, bow case with two bows, a quiver of thirty arrows, and two spare bow strings.[8] Added to the military capability of Arab armies was now a first-rate siege craft and logistics capability.

Like the empire of Rome, the Muslim Empire was a great receptacle in which numerous cultures resided, almost all of which were more sophisticated, worldly, and technologically advanced than the Arabs themselves. The great repository of medical knowledge that the Nestorian monks stored at Jundi-Shapur was now free to flow into the empire and beyond. The Arabs' tolerance for peoples of other faiths, notably Christians and Jews as fellow "peoples of the book," permitted a wide range of contacts with the West through Spain and along the Mediterranean trade routes. Through these contacts, the accumulated medical lore of the Greco-Roman world that was improved and advanced by centuries of contact with Hindu, Chinese, and Persian medical traditions was ready to pour back into the West precisely as Europe was emerging from the Dark Ages of tribalism and beginning to establish the feudal infrastructure upon which the modern states of the area were eventually constructed.

The Arab armies that swept out of Arabia had no medicine at all. Comprising illiterate herdsmen and caravan traders, pre-Islamic Arab society can only be described as primitive. Under Islam, the Quranic precepts prevented the development of any genuinely Arab medicine. It took more than a hundred years to commit the oral tradition of Mohammed to Arabic writing, a task that generated in the Arab a love of learning but only insofar as it related to interpreting and understanding the sacred book. In much the same way that theology and philosophy in the West were regarded as the highest intellectual endeavors, Arabs regarded the study and practice of medicine and other sciences as unworthy earthly pursuits and were left to the conquered peoples of the empire.[9] Arabs who attempted to practice medicine were also limited by the Quran's strictures, which regarded the dead body as unclean. Dissection was forbidden. This restriction led to a poor knowledge of anatomy, as little in the way of clinical investigation of human anatomy was undertaken. As happened in the West, the corrupted Galenic texts became the basis of Arab anatomical studies. Quranic prohibitions against immodesty also made it impossible for Islamic medicine to make any advances in obstetrics, and the refusal of medical practitioners to touch the patient's left hand, regarded as unclean because it was used to wipe oneself, hindered even external medical examination. Denied clinical access to the body, Islamic medicine stressed the use of drugs and other potions to treat illness, while surgery was relegated to secondary status, as it had been in the West.

Some idea of how primitive Arab medicine was in the two centuries between the birth of Mohammed and the establishment of the empire, when contact with more sophisticated medical traditions wrought important changes, can be surmised from an English physician's account written in 1879, or almost four hundred years after medicine in Arabic countries had collapsed.[10] The chronicler recorded that a common medical prescription was prayers from the Quran. Primitive bleeding and purging, often "to the point of extinction," were used to treat fevers and infection. Surgery was butcher surgery, with amputations being accomplished after repeated blows with a chopper, mallet, or short sword and then submersing the limb in boiling pitch or oil to cauterize the stump. Bone setting was crude, and the use of the splint was unknown, with the common result that the limb was often left distorted. Most dentistry was done by traveling barbers.[11] This medicine, then, was what the early soldier of Islam had at his disposal. It was typical of the early Bronze Age, unaided by the advantage of an organized social order that could have systematized and limited its practice.

Without a worthwhile medical tradition of its own and with strong theological restrictions to independent development, it is not surprising that in the Arabic culture, medicine came to be practiced largely by non-Arabs. The tolerance of Islam for other people of the Book made it possible for Christians, Jews, and Persians to dominate the practice of medicine under the empire. Most of these physicians took Arab names and affected Arab dress, but in their thought processes they were the true heirs of the tradition of Jundi-Shapur. The three greatest physicians of the Muslim Empire were all Persians. Rhazes (860–932 CE), who produced ten treatises on medical practice and was a true student of Hippocrates, combined his investigations with Galenic interest for experiment. He was the only example of a quasi-experimental practitioner to emerge under Islam. Haly Abbas (died 994 CE) wrote the *Al-Maliki (Royal Book)*, which was translated into Latin in 1070 CE and became the standard treatise on medicine in the West until the work of Avicenna superseded it. Avicenna's *Canon of Medicine*, a massive tome with sections on surgery, became the definitive medical text of the West from the twelfth to the seventeenth centuries.[12] The influence of Avicenna's work on the West was not all positive, however. His emphasis on deduction instead of clinical observation and investigation reinforced the similar medical tradition in the West for centuries to come. Avicenna's insistence that surgery was less valuable as a branch of medicine than its general practice further reinforced the separation between the two medical branches that the church in Europe had already established.

Meanwhile, by the tenth century, all essential surviving Greek and Roman medical writings had been translated into Arabic. The incalculable value of Rhazes, Haly Abbas, and Avicenna's works was not in any medical innovation, but in their preserving and transmitting the great storehouse of Greco-Roman medical knowledge that had been lost with the collapse of Rome, housed by the Byzantines, brought to Persia by the Nestorians, and finally passed back to the West. Retransmitting this knowledge to the West was the Muslim's most important gift to Western medicine.

In a number of areas, however, the contribution of Islamic medicine was truly original and important. Islamic physicians compiled the most extensive materia medica known at the time. This development naturally followed a medicine that emphasized the application of drugs and compounds over surgery and clinical observation to cure illness. In 970 CE, Abu Mansur Muwaffak compiled the earliest and most important materia medica that Islamic physicians had produced. It lists no fewer than 585 drugs made of 466 vegetable compounds, 75 minerals, and 44 animal compounds prescribed for certain illnesses.[13] In the thirteenth century, Ibn al-Baitar produced another, more comprehensive materia medica comprising 1,400 drugs, at least 300 of which were new to medical knowledge in the West.[14] Much of the Islamic materia medica was of Greek and Roman origin (Dioscorides had been translated into Arabic in Baghdad in 854 CE), but the old collection of remedies had been considerably enhanced by centuries of contact with Persian, Hindu, and Chinese cultures. While the Arabs used many of the same drugs that the Greco-

Romans had for anesthesia, for example, the Islamics seem to have made use of both inhaled anesthetics (hemp fumes) and preoperative compounds to induce sleep before surgery. So important were drugs to the practice of Islamic medicine that the druggist was regarded as a respected member of the medical community. For the first time in history, the medical and pharmacological professions were separated, each with its own professional qualifications and responsibilities.[15]

Another major medical innovation of the Islamics was the formal training and licensing of medical practitioners. As early as 931 CE, a formal educational system for physicians was established in Baghdad. Islamic doctors were trained in universities with attached teaching hospitals and under a mentor and internship system almost identical to the modern system. Graduate physicians were required to pass written and practical examinations, and the hospital chief had to certify their competence in writing. Successful candidates could only practice in their field of training, and a government official who was responsible for public health monitored their performance.[16] Civil authorities specified and enforced a code of behavior for physicians, complete with legal penalties. This system, which the Salerno School in Italy adopted around 1140, represented the first formal process of training and licensing of medical practitioners that the West had seen since the Roman era.[17]

The Muslim system of formal education stimulated the construction of medical libraries that were larger than anything the world had seen in a millennium. The great library of Alexandria, which Christian zealots destroyed in the second century CE, was reputed to have contained 300,000 volumes. By contrast, the library at Tripoli in Lebanon contained *3 million* volumes before the Crusaders burned it in 1109. The Fatimid library in Egypt held 2 million volumes, and the library in Cordova, Spain, contained more than 600,000 medical books.[18] While due credit must be given to the Christian monasteries of Europe that also built libraries of great value, for their sheer size, scope, and diversity of collections none could match the great medical libraries of the Islamic world.

Perhaps the most important contribution of Islamic physicians was the construction of hospitals. The Muslims were the first to establish medical training and teaching within a modern university–teaching hospital setting. These hospitals were all built on the model of the great university and hospital at Jundi-Shapur in Persia, with the first Islamic hospital established in Damascus in 706 CE. The word for hospital in Arabic is *bimaristan,* a Persian loan meaning "a place for sick people."[19] It is important to note that the motivation for building these institutions was primarily religious and not medical. The Quran requires that the wealthy and powerful look after the poor and weak, and wealthy benefactors seeking to live their faith founded and funded the hospitals. The Quranic impulse was further reflected in the fact that the poor were treated without charge and given free prescriptions, and discharged patients received money to help them survive during their recovery.

The Arab hospitals were modern in design and practice. Because Quranic law forbade women to appear unveiled before the opposite sex, the typical hospital had two separate sections, one for each sex, that were furnished with nursing staffs and porters of their patients' respective genders. There is no evidence, though, of female doctors. Each of the hospital's two main sections was arranged into separate wards based on the type of disease treated and was further subdivided into subsections to segregate patients by the type of illness they suffered. Some attempts were made to confine certain diseases to special clinics.[20]

As in modern hospitals, Islamic hospitals had both an inpatient and outpatient department, and outpatient receptions were confined to certain days of the week. Inpatients were admitted and assigned to special areas by type of disease, and each ward had from one to three physicians who specialized in that disease. Visiting staff members also took turns of duty, during which they were required to remain available within hospital grounds. A typical duty shift required the doctor to spend two days and two nights each week in the hospital.[21]

Given the highly developed hospital system and the Quranic directive to provide care for the sick, Islamic medicine developed a completely new form of medical care: the traveling hospital. These mobile hospitals were transported by pack animals to areas where epidemics raged or in outlying areas where a need for medical attention arose. These hospitals were a permanent part of the overall medical care system in that permanent travel routes and some schedules were established, and doctors and other personnel attached to these hospitals functioned on a regular or even a career basis.[22] These hospitals were equipped with medicines, instruments, tents, and a complete staff of physicians and orderlies, but the quality of the assigned medical personnel might have been lower than that found in the fixed hospitals.[23] These mobile hospitals also served the prisons and, of course, the military. In one description, a mobile military hospital was transported to the battlefield by forty camels.[24]

Formally established military medical care for Islamic armies seems to have come about somewhat late in the imperial period. The first evidence of any military care emerges in the later half of the tenth century (950?) in a medical text written by Abul Qasim, who states that his chapter on surgery was based on his experience as a surgeon attached to the army.[25] The stimulus for providing medical care to the troops probably arose as a consequence of Islamic armies' contact with the Byzantines who, as noted, had the most highly developed military medical service of the period. Except for the mobile military hospitals, we know little about the structure of the medical service in Islamic armies. Drawing upon the descriptions of battle wounds and their treatment found in the works of Rhazes and Abul Qasim, it seems reasonable to infer that trained physicians accompanied the armies and provided medical care on a routine basis.[26] It is also likely that the ribats had medical staffs attached to them. There is, however, no evidence of a permanent military medical corps that trained its own people and organized its own supplies. Instead, it seems, the armies drew upon the highly developed resources of the civilian medical establishment in times of war. Except for the usual hygienic practices commonly found in military camps in almost all armies except those of the West, we know little of any permanent military medical structure for Islamic armies.[27]

The quality of military medical care seems to have been at least as good as what the Byzantines provided to their armies. While surgery had a low reputation in the West, and although Avicenna thought surgery to be of lower status than the general practice of medicine, surgery remained a respectable and valued branch of medicine throughout the Islamic period. Interestingly, the frequency with which amputations were performed suggests as well that the practice of ligature was not lost to Islamic physicians. The use of cautery with pitch or oil suggests standard Galenic surgical practice was also well established. Most important, the deadly doctrine of natural infection does not appear to have taken root in Islamic medicine. The presence of mobile military hospitals would also have given Islamic military medical care a significant advantage insofar as trained physicians were available to stop blood loss and prevent shock. In the main, then, Islamic military medicine may have been as effective as that practiced by the Byzantine armies of the same period.

On the one hand, analysis of military medical care in the Islamic period leads one to conclude that Islamic medicine was not as revolutionary and innovative as it was perceived to be in the West at the time. The erroneous Western perception resulted from the general decline in medical knowledge that accompanied the Middle Ages. On the other hand, because the Islamics were the heirs to the medical tradition bequeathed by the Nestorians and Persians at Jundi-Shapur, most of the sound military medical practices of the Greco-Roman period were commonly utilized with generally good results. To be sure, the religious strictures of the Quran retarded any independent development of anatomy and surgery, but religion never had the devastating impact on medical science of the Islamic Empire that it had in the West. By the time of the Crusades, the wounded in Islamic armies still had a better chance of surviving their wounds than did those in Crusader armies.[28]

The Middle Ages

The period of the High Middle Ages (800–1453 CE) was a time of violent transition that began at the end of the Dark Ages and concluded with the Renaissance. When it began, Europe was still attempting, after years of barbarization, to reestablish an imperium along Roman lines, the dream that drove Charlemagne. When it ended, the idea of an imperium was dead and replaced by the quilt-like pattern of the national state system that has survived to this day. The Hundred Years' War (1337–1453 CE) endowed these proto-national entities with national kings who were capable of raising national armies and who could overcome the decentralizing effects of feudalism by establishing strong, centralized administrative structures that were loyal to the kings and gave practical effect to royal commands. The result was the emergence of national identities that superseded any claims to imperial or transnational loyalties, that is, to anyone except the monarch as head of the new national state. In 1453, the Byzantine Empire, the last competitor for the legacy of the Roman imperium as a model for Western political organization, fell to the Ottoman Turks.

During the seven hundred years of the High Middle Ages, Europe was wracked by dynastic struggles, renewed invasions from outside its borders, brigandage, guerrilla wars, and national conflicts. The Viking invasions of the ninth century added such havoc to an already chaotic state of affairs that the church conceived of the First Crusade (to be followed by seven others) as a mechanism for deflecting the feudal combatants' warlike spirit toward targets outside Europe. For seven centuries, Europe knew little respite from the ravages of war and destruction.

The centralizing efforts of Charlemagne (742–814 CE) resulted in the solidification of a new feudal order marked by extreme decentralization in all political, economic, social, and military functions. The next seven centuries may best be defined by the constant struggle between the forces of centralization, led by would-be national monarchs, against the forces of decentralization that characterized feudalism as a form of societal organization. In the end, the forces of centralization won out but proved unequal to the task of reestablishing any form of imperial order encompassing national identity and loyalty. Europe was giving birth to the nation-state.

The effect of this state of affairs on military developments was gradual but certain. At the beginning of the period, armies were collections of feudal vassals serving for short periods in the wars of their lords. Eventually, however, the aristocratic knightly classes could not satisfy the demand for manpower. The kings turned to recruiting "men-at-arms" from the lower social orders, bringing into being national armies that were independent of the landed aristocracy. With the exception of the crossbow and longbow, weapon development was marginal, and the introduction of plate armor for the horse-borne warrior became a symbol of the triumph of the defense over the offense. The period witnessed the age of fortification in which massive castles and fortified towns sprang up all over Europe. The cavalry remained supreme until the threat of missiles fired by bow and crossbow on their formations forced them to dismount, heralding a return to the use of infantry.[29] The military experience of the Crusades forced European armies to develop rudimentary logistical skills, but they never achieved any real level of effectiveness. The introduction of gunpowder and the cannon, both innovations of enormous importance, had only a limited immediate effect on warfare. It required almost two centuries to turn these technological developments into truly significant killing implements.

The Middle Ages produced little in the way of medical advancement. Although the church had removed its traditional ban on dissection in medical schools, the technique was never used to advance anatomical knowledge.[30] Rather, dissection was seen as an impressive way for the faculty to demonstrate its medical knowledge to students.[31] Medicine remained in the grip of deductive methods of reasoning; consequently, experimentation and clinical experience were little used in the development of clinical treatments. Establishing medical schools at Salerno and Montpellier in Europe did little to reverse this trend, and the still-enforced harsh penalties for causing a patient's death by surgery kept medical practice in a passive mode in which poultices and drugs were preferred to surgical intervention. To curtail what the church saw as the negative effects of medical practice upon monastic orders, it all but outlawed clerical physicians from practicing surgery. It was left to the barber-physicians, some of whom were marginally competent, but most were dangerous quacks whose activities gave surgery an even worse name and solidified its separation from general medicine for almost four hundred years.[32] Under these circumstances, coupled with the generally decentralized organization of the armies of the day, it is hardly surprising that military medicine remained stagnant.

Under feudalism, the vassals within the lord's realm raised armies. Large armies were coalitions of forces, each serving under their local commanders. In this sense, these armies formalized the old, Germanic tribal military structure. Each vassal was responsible for providing not only the men but also their weapons, equipment, horses, and food as there was centralized commissariat to provide for the army as a whole. The warrior aristocrats could afford to pay a doctor to attend them on military campaign, but there was no medical service either for the army as a whole or for the men within the vassal's troop. Few of the civilian society's barber-surgeons and quacks attended an army in the field because there was no money to be made from treating common soldiers. The aristocrats would have nothing to do with these barbers in any case, preferring instead the medical attention of the internist. With no permanent medical personnel in the army, it is not surprising that it was left to camp followers and women, often wives, who accompanied the army to provide what medical attention the soldier needed. Further, no system existed for evacuating the wounded or transporting them from the battlefield to places of care.

The Crusades (1096–1272 CE) brought about some changes in military medical care. For the most part, the Crusades involved large, unorganized caravans of soldiers, civilian businessmen, people looking for a new start, and, at least in the early days, pilgrims. There was no military organization whatsoever. The formation of the Knights Hospitallers to provide medical care to the sick and wounded as a matter of Christian duty did much to establish hospitals where surviving wounded or disease-stricken soldiers could be brought for medical attention. Since these hospitals were open to anyone, even the common soldier received medical care within their walls.[33] Accounts of the Crusades also record aristocrats being treated for battle injuries by their personal attending physicians and the common practice of evacuating wounded knights on litters or upon their long triangular shields. One searches in vain, however, for any sort of organization that delivered medical care to the wounded on a regular basis.

A portrait of military medical care during this period emerges from the Romantic epics of the time. From the *chansons de geste* (songs of honor, or epic poems), the *Le Morte d'Arthur,* and the *Chanson de Roland,* there emerges a portrait of medical care for the soldier similar to that found in the *Iliad.* The wounded knight was laid upon the ground and given a stimulating "wound-drink" to relieve faintness, oil or wine was poured into his wounds, and hemorrhage and pain were relieved by herbs or wound sucking. Various charms or prayers were said over the wound, and the pulse was checked to determine the seriousness of the knight's condition. If possible, the soldier was moved into the shade or some other comfortable spot, where he would either recover by his own means or die.[34] Homer would have probably recognized the scene as applying to his generation, and it might be said as well that the medical treatment was just as useless.

During the Crusades, the poor state of military medical care is reflected in the filthy conditions of military camps. The art of field hygiene and sanitation had been lost completely. The disease figures for the Crusader armies demonstrate a lack of basic knowledge of contagion. In 1098 CE, a Christian army laid siege to Antioch. Disease killed so many besiegers that the dead were too numerous to bury. Of the seven thousand horses provided for the cavalry, five thousand succumbed to disease.[35] During the Second Crusade, famine and disease had reduced Louis VII's army of 100,000 men to a mere 5,000 by the time it reached the Holy Land.[36] In 1190 CE, as Saladin besieged Acre, a pestilence broke out among the Crusader army. The Crusaders died at a rate of 200 men a day.[37] In the Fifth Crusade (1218), the Crusaders besieged Damietta. Pestilence and disease carried off a fifth of the army in less than a month.[38] The Crusaders' disorganized military structure and poor medical knowledge consistently combined to wreak havoc through disease on army after army over a seven-hundred-year period.

It was not until 1419 CE that the terrible ravages of disease were finally addressed by rudimentary regulations on camp hygiene. In that year Henry V published in his *Ordinances of War* the directive that officers were to ensure that the offal of beasts slaughtered for food was to be buried.[39] Twenty years later, an English king issued orders that water first be "cleansed and pourged by boyllynge."[40] In 1498 CE a tract on camp hygiene extracted from the writings of Arnold of Villanova recommended that drinking water be tested before troops were allowed to consume it and that slit trenches be located outside the camp.[41] There is no evidence, however, that any of these regulations were implemented on a regular basis or that any officers were specifically charged with overseeing their implementation.

During the Hundred Years' War, Jean Froissart recorded that it was common practice for the French army to remove its wounded from the battlefield to a nearby house for dressing wounds, but the manner of treatment was still primitive.[42] Doctors and surgeons were rare during the conflict, and there were only primitive efforts to establish medical treatment for the troops. Twenty years after the Battle of Hastings (1066 CE), the *Doomsday Book* recorded the presence of two military surgeons, and in 1300 CE Prince Edward of England invaded Scotland and was accompanied by seven medical practitioners, including the king's personal physician, two assistants, a king's surgeon, two assistants, and a simple surgeon.[43] While it has been argued that this cadre constituted the first attempt since the Roman era to provide a standing medical service for an army, by 1346 CE the muster of the English army listed no medical personnel at all.[44]

Other instances of physicians attending the army appear in the next two centuries. In 1415 CE at the Battle of Agincourt, King Henry V was accompanied by a physician, a surgeon, and twelve assistants.[45] In 1470 CE Edward IV of England in his campaign against Louis XI of France was attended by a chief physician, two personal body physicians, a surgeon, and thirteen assistant barber-surgeons.[46] The barber-surgeons probably provided some medical care to the soldiery, but there is no evidence that this occurred.

Only two bright spots in providing medical care to the soldiery appeared in the long, dark night of the Middle Ages. After the Battle of Laupen in 1339 CE, the Swiss cantons regularly voted monies to provide for the care of the wounded and their dependents. Individual cantons also engaged the regular use of barber-surgeons to attend the wounded after the battle.[47] In France in the 1470s, Charles the Bold placed a surgeon in each company of one hundred lancers and their attendants, thus providing one surgeon for every eight hundred men.[48] Charles's actions are recognized as the first instance in his period of a commander providing medical care to his troops as well as to his officers.[49] During the Thirty Years' War (1618–1648), Gustavus Adolphus also provided similar medical facilities for his troops.[50]

Not until the late 1400s is there any evidence of a regular medical service in a European army, and then it was found only in Spain. In the wars of Ferdinand and Isabella against the Moors, the Spanish kings copied the Islamic mobile military medical hospitals and introduced them to the Spanish armies. At the siege of Alora (1484) and Baza (1489), Spanish forces were provided with six large hospital tents to treat the wounded. Special covered wagons with beds were used to transport the sick and wounded in the first example of an ambulance service in medieval armies.[51] Like the Islamic model, Spanish hospitals were mobile; employed regular physicians, surgeons, and attendants; and contained furniture and medicine cabinets. Following the siege of Malaga (1487), some four hundred wagons carrying the sick and wounded entered the city.[52] The Spanish use of mobile military hospitals can be attributed to the strong Islamic presence in Spain for more than six hundred years, during which time the Spanish had adequate opportunity to observe the Islamic medical practice. For the rest of Europe, where Islamic influence was much less present, however, military medical care never attained the level that it did in Spain.

The period from the collapse of the Roman Empire in the West to the Renaissance can only be described as a low point in the development of military medicine. The long empirical medical tradition of the West culminating in the establishment of the Roman military medical service went into eclipse for the next thousand years. With the exception of the Byzantines and the Islamics, who preserved and practiced the old medicine of the Greeks and Romans, medical care of any type in the West regressed to levels not seen since the Bronze Age. The collapse of any central political authority made it impossible to establish any institutional mechanisms for preserving, teaching, and transmitting medical knowledge, while the Christian church's imposition of a strongly superstitious and philosophical approach to the world led to a turning away from the material world and a denigration of observation and empiricism as a guide to knowledge. The result was a medical catastrophe in which the treatment of disease and battle wounds was largely ineffective.

The armies of the period also reflected the general organizational chaos of their respective larger societies. Consequently, the experiences of the battlefield, which in almost every culture for four thousand years had spurred the advancement of clinical medical technique, now produced no valuable knowledge to care for the wounded soldier. Theological and social norms relegated the clinical practitioner's role to such a low status that his few skills were never brought to bear on the treatment of battle casualties. Almost three hundred years passed before the armies of Europe began to offer a level of military medical care that approached what had been available to the legions of Rome and Byzantium. In that interim, millions of soldiers succumbed needlessly to wounds that would have been effectively treated in an earlier age.

Notes

1. The tolerance of Islam for other religions became more attractive to the subjects of the Byzantine and Persian Empires after the imperial authorities' rigorous persecution of heretical Christian sects. Many persecuted Christians sought refuge in Islam and willingly supported and joined the invading Muslim armies. Richard A. Gabriel, *Muhammad: Islam's First Great General* (Norman: University of Oklahoma Press, 2007), 18–19.
2. Laffont, *Ancient Art of Warfare*, 179; and Gabriel, *Muhammad*, 19–22.
3. Newark, *The Barbarians*, 86–87.
4. Gabriel, *Muhammad*, chapter 3, "Arab Warfare." For an analysis of Muhammad's insurgency and military campaigns, see Richard A. Gabriel, "The Warrior Prophet," *Military History Quarterly* 19, no. 4 (Summer 2007): 6–15.
5. Ibid., 207–19, for al-Walid's reforms and his conduct of military campaigns.
6. For an analysis of the military's use of the camel compared to that of the horse in desert warfare, see Gabriel, *Muhammad*, 36–42.
7. Laffont, *Ancient Art of Warfare*, 180. In the same way that Roman military forts sometimes became major cities, the Islamic military garrisons sometimes became major cities. The ribat in Morocco, for example, became the capital, Rabat.

8. Newark, *The Barbarians*, 96.
9. Elgood, *Medical History of Persia*, 261–62. The nine sacred Muslim sciences that emerged as a consequence of the Quran being put into writing were exegesis, criticism, apostolic tradition, grammar, jurisprudence, theology, lexicography, rhetoric, and literature. Left to foreigners were medicine, philosophy, geometry, astronomy, music, magic, and alchemy.
10. Garrison, *Introduction to the History of Medicine*, 147–48.
11. Ibid.
12. Maurice Atiyeh, "Arab Hospitals in History," *King Faisal Specialist Hospital Medical Journal* 2, no. 2 (1982): 122. The two outstanding translators of Arabic material into Latin were Constantinus Africanus (1020–1087 CE), who worked at the monastery of Monte Cassino, and Gerard of Cremona (1114–1187 CE), who worked in Toledo. Ackerknecht, *Short History of Medicine*, 85.
13. Garrison, *Introduction to the History of Medicine*, 133.
14. Ibid.
15. Elgood, *A Medical History of Persia*, 174.
16. The official charged with overseeing the public food, water, and pharmacological supply was called a *muhtasib*.
17. Ackerknecht, *Short History of Medicine*, 92. The regulations were promulgated by King Roger II of Sicily in 1140 CE and prescribed state examinations for those who wanted to practice medicine. The previous Roman medical licensing system had collapsed in the third century.
18. Atiyeh, "Arab Hospitals in History," 125.
19. Elgood, *A Medical History of Persia*, 174.
20. See ibid., 176–78, for a description of the Arab hospital.
21. Ibid.
22. Ibid., 175. See also Reuben Levy, *A Baghdad Chronicle* (Cambridge, UK: Cambridge University Press, 1929), 212.
23. Elgood, *A Medical History of Persia*, 174. It may be doubted that the quality of physicians available to the mobile hospitals was of the same caliber as those in the prestigious fixed hospitals located in the empire's major cities. It is likely that mostly apprentices and the recent graduates of medical schools staffed the mobile hospitals.
24. Atiyeh, "Arab Hospitals in History," 122.
25. Weston P. Chamberlain, "History of Military Medicine and Its Contributions to Science," *Boston Medical and Surgical Journal*, April 1917, 237. The Arabs produced only one great surgeon, Abul Qasim (1013–1106 CE). Ackerknecht, *Short History of Medicine*, 84.
26. For a good analysis of the chapters in Rhazes and Albucasis as they pertain to military medicine, see Garrison, *Notes on the History of Military Medicine*, 82.

27. The sections of Rhazes dealing with military hygiene in the camp have been translated by Frölich and are quoted in English in ibid., 83.

28. A comparison of medicine of the Crusaders with Islamic medicine of the period is found in Piers D. Mitchell, *Medicine in the Crusades: Warfare, Wounds, and the Medieval Surgeon* (New York: Cambridge University Press, 2005).

29. Another important factor in the return of infantry to the battlefield was the rediscovery by the Swiss of the disciplined pike phalanx, whose leveled weapons effectively neutralized the mounted knights' cavalry charge.

30. For a detailed analysis of the restrictions and intentions of the various church documents prohibiting the practice of surgery by clerics during this period, see Darrel W. Amundsen, "Medieval Canon Law on Medical and Surgical Practice by the Clergy," *Bulletin of the History of Medicine* 52 (1978): 22–44. Amundsen argues that the church had intended to prohibit regular clergy from the practice while exempting secular clergy from the restrictions. He does acknowledge, however, that the effect of these edicts was to drive the practice of surgery into the hands of the untrained.

31. Ackerknecht, *Short History of Medicine*, 90.

32. "Surgery was now left to barbers, bath-keepers, hangmen, sow-gelders, and mountebanks and quacks of every description." Ibid., 89. See also Marie-Christine Pouchelle, *The Body and Surgery in the Middle Ages*, trans. Rosemary Morris (New Brunswick, NJ: Rutgers University Press, 1990).

33. An excellent analysis of the military hospital movement during the Crusades is found in Edgar Eskine Hume, "Medical Work of the Knights Hospitallers of St. John of Jerusalem," paper delivered before the New York Academy of Medicine, 1936. One of the few positive achievements of medicine during the Middle Ages was the movement to found hospitals. By 1200 CE a network of hospitals covered most of Europe. As noted earlier, these hospitals were not primarily medical institutions but philanthropic institutions offering "hospitality" to the old, disabled, and homeless. It would take another century before hospitals acquired their role as medical institutions. Ackerknecht, *Short History of Medicine*, 92–93.

34. G. M. Gould and W. L. Pyle, "King Arthur's Medicine," *Johns Hopkins Hospital Bulletin* 7 (1897): 239–46.

35. Reginald Hargreaves, "Ally of Defeat," *The Practitioner* 202 (May 1960): 714.

36. Ibid.

37. Carey P. McCord, "Scurvy as an Occupational Disease," *Journal of Occupational Medicine* 13, no. 12 (December 1971): 587.

38. Ibid.

39. Hargreaves, "Long Road to Military Hygiene," 440.

40. Ibid.

41. Garrison, *Notes on the History of Military Medicine*, 95.

42. Ibid.

43. Chamberlain, "History of Military Medicine," 237.

44. Ibid.

45. Ibid.

46. John F. Fulton, "Medicine, Warfare, and History," *Journal of the American Medical Association* 153, no. 5 (October 1953): 428.

47. Ibid., 427.

48. Ibid.

49. Ibid.

50. Ibid.

51. Garrison, *Notes on the History of Military Medicine*, 95.

52. Ibid., 96.

12

MILITARY MEDICINE IN
THE ANCIENT WORLD

This book has focused on the development of military medicine in the ancient world, a world that began four thousand years before the birth of Christ and ended with the collapse of the feudal order in Europe in the middle of the fifteenth century. The year 1453 CE marked the end of the ancient period when the Ottoman Turks' forces finally overran and destroyed the Byzantine Empire and captured the city of Constantinople itself. The last continuous cultural link with the empire of Rome was finally severed, and with it the last contiguous cultural tradition of the ancient world came to an end. The Ottomans' use of artillery cannon to breach the walls of Constantinople was a portent of future developments in warfare, a symbol of a genuine sea change in military technology that would shape warfare for the next six centuries.

When the Hundred Years' War ended in Europe in the same year, the last remnants of the feudal order that Charlemagne had established six centuries earlier finally collapsed. The central feudal idea of a commonwealth of Christian nations united within a common political, transnational order and bound by shared interests and cultural, political, religious, and social institutions broke apart on the shoals of emerging states, each grounded within its own national identity, demarcated by clear geographic boundaries, and ruled by national monarchs who recognized no earthly constraints upon their prerogatives. Feudal armies gave way to genuine national armies fired by national loyalties and supported by national treasuries, new instruments that monarchs used to press the interests of their states. A new age of weaponry was also dawning as the muscle-powered weapons of the past slowly but surely gave way to weapons powered by chemical explosion. A military technology that had remained unchanged in its essentials and killing power for more than two thousand years was on the brink of a technological revolution that would eventually change warfare forever. The ancient world was dying a slow but inevitable death.

People living in the modern era are unaware of just how remarkable that ancient world truly was and how much the modern world owes to it. The period between 4000 BCE and 400 CE was among the most creative eras of human development. Many of the social, economic, political, and military structures that undergird modern institutions and technology are innovations that the ancients bequeathed to us. In all forms of social development, it is always easier to improve an existing structure, practice, institution, or idea than it is to invent it in the first place. The ancients were truly inventors in many areas of human endeavor.[1] Among their most important innovations was writing, first in pictographs, then in more advanced ideogramic phonetic forms such as cuneiform and hieroglyphics, and later in alphabetic script. To place this remarkable invention in perspective, it is only necessary to remember that humans have existed in their present biological form for at least two hundred thousand years, but they have been able to write for fewer than six thousand of those years.

Humans of the ancient period may have evolved through a complex change in brain function that made modern empiricism possible and altered the way in which our intellectual processes work. Prior to the introduction of written text language circa 700 BCE, the human brain seems to have functioned in a highly bicameral fashion in which right lobe functions were dominant. An analysis of thousands of portraits of humans and animals prior to 650 BCE shows that the great majority of them faced to the viewer's left, an indication of right hemisphere brain dominance. Portraits drawn *after* the introduction of written text language show the sitters facing to the viewer's right, indicating the emergence of left hemisphere dominance. Early Greek writing appears to have been genuinely transitional in that it required both hemispheres to function simultaneously. This early writing began from left to right, dropped down a line, and moved right to left, working in the same fashion as a computer printer.

As portrayed in the *Iliad,* the *Legend of Gilgamesh,* and the Bible, the ancients' ability to hear voices or talk to the gods might suggest that their brain functions may have been more bicameral than those of modern humans. While the evidence is far from conclusive, if this hypothesis is so, then the ancient world may have given birth to one of the most significant biological changes that humans have ever experienced, a change that resulted in left lobe dominance of the brain. Left-sided dominance is absolutely required for the birth of writing, mathematics, logic, medicine, and systematic science—all essential ingredients to achieve the advanced technology upon which the modern world is based.[2]

The ancient period witnessed the birth of society itself. Until the fourth millennium BCE, humans lived in small bands of hunter-gatherers, a form of social organization that made sophisticated social, economic, political, military, and scientific development impossible. The first large-scale human social orders emerged in the ancient period and were based on stable agriculture. Before the invention of agricultural societies, there were no priesthoods, codified religions, public bureaucrats, political rulers, scribes, merchants, farmers, professional soldiers, armies, libraries, medical schools, and a thousand other socially differentiated roles and institutions so familiar to modern humans.

These early societies were much more than primitive social prototypes, for in the same period humans invented genuine cities. In the fourth millennium BCE, the city of Uruk in Sumer enclosed an area of 5.5 square miles within its city walls, or more than twice the size of ancient Athens, four times the size of ancient Jerusalem at the time of Christ, and almost as large as the city of Rome in 100 CE. By the third millennium BCE, the cities of Sumer regularly incorporated thirty thousand to forty thousand inhabitants. Along with the large concentrations of inhabitants came the invention of water supplies, bridges, temples, aqueducts, sewers, running water, dikes, and other elements of a modern urban infrastructure.

It was in the ancient period that the first political institutions emerged along with the first modern bureaucracies, complete with the written records required for effective governance. Indeed, ancient forms of social organization reached such tremendous heights that they remained the prototypes of human social organization until the birth of the modern nation-state in the fifteenth century CE. Moreover, the emergence of the imperium permitted the ancients to organize and operate political, social, and economic units on a scale far greater than any of the nation-states of even the eighteenth century achieved. The modern nation-states have their roots in the imperial national units of Assyria and Rome and are heavily indebted to these civilizations for developing the initial means to govern them.

The ancient world also gave birth to the prototypes of modern science and medicine. Mathematics, chemistry, astronomy, medicine, architecture, and engineering all began in the ancient period. The institution of war itself first emerged during this time, and ancient soldiers invented professional armies whose size, complexity, operational capability, equipment, and destructive power were greater than anything armies of the modern era produced until the American Civil War. With the exception of the rifle, the military engineers of the ancient world invented and refined the prototype of every modern weapon that the soldier used until the eighteenth century CE. Modern tactics are simply refinements of ancient commanders' innovations, and no army in the West could match the logistics capabilities of Roman armies until the time of Napoleon. After that, it required the invention of the railroad to move an army faster than a Roman legion could move. From the fifth century until at least the eighteenth century, the armies of the West regularly carried out operations at a lower level of military proficiency than had many of the armies of the ancient period.

Ancient armies also invented the prototypes of the modern soldier's combat equipment: helmet, body armor, boots, and backpack. Until the nineteenth century, even the killing power of combat weapons was below that of ancient armies. No weapon could fire as rapidly, over as long a distance, and with greater accuracy than the composite bow until the introduction of the Prussian needle gun in 1841. Napoleon's artillery fired over shorter ranges than Philip II of Macedon's torsion-powered catapults, and the eight- to ten-pound cannonball used throughout the American Civil War was lighter by a factor of ten than Roman stone artillery shot. The Roman repeating field gun could fire four to five rounds a minute, a rate of artillery fire not matched until the appearance of the breech-loading cannon and one-piece shell after the Civil War.

This level of military proficiency was rooted in a much more important invention of the ancients, namely, war itself. It is sobering to recall that prior to the fourth millennium BCE, there is precious little evidence of any sort of war conducted on any scale. The emergence of war seems tied to the invention of agriculture, which made congregating large populations within cities possible. This arrangement, in turn, increased the opportunities for social differentiation that led directly to the emergence of the standing army as a major institution of human society. To the Greeks, modern soldiers owe the myth of military heroism, a product of the particular sociology of the Greek city-states. The belief that only war provided the opportunity for the full development of human virtues found its way into Western civilization via Rome and influenced the way humans thought about war for the next fifteen hundred years. The military medicine of the ancient armies, especially those of Rome and the Hindus, was superior to anything the soldier received in the West until the nineteenth century CE. No army of the West utilized a military medical service equal to that of the Roman armies until the Civil War. No antibiotic was more effective than the honey paste that the Egyptian army of the first millennium BCE concocted until the invention of penicillin, nor was any antiseptic more effective than the Roman's acetum until Lister pioneered carbolic acid's application as a surgical antiseptic. The evidence seems conclusive that the military doctors of the ancient world were far more successful in preventing and dealing with infection than any physicians until at least the nineteenth century.

The origins and development of military medicine and the establishment of a formal military medical corps have strong roots in the military organizations of the ancient world. Medicine is a product of relatively complex civilizations, and military medicine is a product of sophisticated military organization. In the developmental scheme of things, medicine appeared first in those ancient civilizations whose societies were sufficiently large, articulated, and centrally organized to permit the advancement of specially organized social structures that could investigate, learn, record, and transmit knowledge about injury and disease. Although it is probable that humans organized in hunter-gatherer social orders included shamans who claimed special knowledge of the causes and cures of illness and disease, the emergence of medicine as a coherent body of knowledge and object of clinical practice could never have materialized in these loose and transitory social structures. The organization of knowledge requires stable social organization as well.

As best we know, the medical professions of the ancient world's earliest social orders were centered around the new priesthoods. This association is not surprising in light of the essentially magical and religious explanations for illness and disease that have accompanied humans since earliest times. Once the transition from mobile clans to stable social orders was achieved, the priesthoods became more organizationally defined and entrenched in the new societies, and quite naturally they continued and expanded upon traditional explanations for medical concerns. It could have happened no other way until a larger experiential base of information permitted the conceptualization of alternative explanations for illness and disease.

Medicine owes much to these early priestly castes, for they first organized, however primitively, the search for knowledge into medical matters. Equally important, these priests' ability to write permitted the recording and transmission of medical knowledge as it gradually accumulated through the ages. Without their transcribing this information, medical schools and the establishment of medical traditions for use by future generations would have been impossible.

The development of an army's military medicine depended crucially on the state of that army's organizational development. The degree of military organizational development, in turn, was determined by the frequency of war that the various early states had to endure. In Egypt, for example, which was relatively isolated from foreign threats for almost two thousand years, military organizational development remained primitive; thus, its military medicine developed more slowly than in other armies of the period. By contrast, the city-states of Sumer were at war for almost two thousand years. Consequently, the first evidence of an army providing medical care to its soldiers on the battlefield is found in Sumer. When it came to the development of military medicine, necessity was the mother of invention.

This same pattern reoccurred throughout the ancient world. Where warfare was frequent and armies highly developed, military medicine advanced in a corresponding manner. Thus, on the one hand, the constant warfare among the Hindu states of the Indian subcontinent produced a strongly articulated military medical service, along with significant advances in clinical treatment of the wounded. The same may be said for the Romans. Classical Greece, on the other hand, represented a civilization where warfare among city-states was both less frequent and less threatening to the survival of these states. The result was that military medical care remained at a comparatively low level. Not surprising, the emergence of a military medical service as a cultural artifact of the social and military orders of the ancient world depended heavily on the frequency and nature of warfare that the social order itself had to endure.

The dominant cultural perspective of the early societies also influenced the development of military medicine. The ancient Hebrews, for example, lived in a theocratic society whose dominant cultural perspectives led to a passive view of humans' ability to deal with illnesses, which were seen as punishments from god. Although the Bible is full of accounts of battles and wars, there is no evidence that military medicine was present on the battlefield. A similar situation occurred in ancient Greece and early Rome, where the cultural ideals of stoic endurance, courage, and personal glory militated against the development of military medicine within their armies. The cultural values of the Persian Empire, with their emphasis on humans trapped between the larger forces of universal good and evil, led to a similar failure to develop military medicine.

The level of the armies' organizational sophistication also played an important role in whether and to what degree a state made progress in military medicine. As in modern times, the overall level of military sophistication largely determined the ability of armies to provide certain capabilities. The armies of Rome, the Hindu states, and Assyria were the most highly developed armies of their day, and they all operated highly sophisticated military medical services. The small citizen armies of Greece, the tribally organized armies of Persia and the early Middle Ages in Europe, and the armies of feudal Europe all failed to establish military medical services of any consequence.

It is important to note that the level of organizational sophistication of the various armies of the ancient world did not follow any consistent pattern. Some of the earliest armies, notably Sumer and Assyria, were far more developed and articulated than the armies of Greece, Persia, Islam, and the European feudal order that came later. The same, of course, can be said for their respective military medical services. The lack of any coherent pattern of longitudinal development in military organizational forms is important, for it speaks to the low level of cultural and technological transfer between societies that characterized the ancient period. While the modern world experiences a rapid pace of informational and technological imitation and transfer, it rarely occurred in the ancient world. Customs, habits, practices, and organizational forms often persisted long after they had lost any functional value.

This constancy explains, for example, why we find so few examples of the transfer of medical knowledge from one society to another, even though two societies might have been in cultural contact for long periods. The extensive contacts of Egyptian and Greek medicine, for example, produced few examples of transferred medical knowledge. Instead, Egyptian medicine continued its decline into mysticism for almost three hundred years, only taking cognizance of the Greek empirical tradition after Alexander the Great's conquest of Egypt. Likewise, Persia's extensive connections with Greek medical empirics had no impact at all on Persian medicine until after the collapse of the empire. Even Assyria's common medical and cultural tradition with the earlier Sumerians could not prevent the Assyrian descent into medical magic. Even the early Hebrews' close contact with Egyptian medicine produced not a single change in the primitive Hebraic view of medicine. A society's willingness to adopt new ideas is a complex process that is highly dependent on numerous variables that go far beyond the degree to which the proposed change can be shown to be functional. For most of human history, societies have shown a marked reluctance to adopt new ideas regardless of the source from which they sprung. Our understanding of the ancient world and the evolution of military medicine is enhanced if we remember that the rapid pace of informational and cultural exchange and transfer to which we are accustomed is a modern phenomenon indeed.

The degree of separation between a social order's secular and religious authorities is another important variable in understanding how military medicine evolved throughout the ancient world. With few exceptions, the states of the ancient world had relatively close relationships with the church. Within this general limitation, however, two patterns emerged. A number of states, such as Egypt, Israel, and those of feudal Europe, reveal a pattern in which religious sectors of society were dominant in most important respects. Other states, such as Sumer, Assyria, and Rome, reflected the opposite model in which secular power was dominant. In Sumer and Assyria this predominance was achieved relatively early in their history, while in the Hindu states and feudal Europe religious interference in secular affairs ended relatively late.

It seems no accident that those societies with strong secular authorities capable of controlling the priesthoods or relegating them largely to religious functions also produced the most organizationally sophisticated armies and the most developed military medical services. In Sumer, for example, the king was able to separate his secular powers from religious interference very early. In doing so, the Sumerian kings were able to obtain first claim on all social resources for prosecuting their wars, including control over military medical assets. Thus, clinical medical practitioners served on the battlefields in Sumer even though the medical profession itself remained in the grip of the priesthood. By contrast, during the Middle Ages the Christian church exercised control over secular affairs and prevented the kings from using medical resources on the battlefield. It seems that no societies whose secular orders remained subordinate to religious influences succeeded in developing functional military medical institutions.

The tension between secular and religious authorities as a factor in the development of military medicine is clear enough insofar as it represents a struggle for control over material resources. Perhaps more important, however, was the tension between religious authorities and medical science for control of the body of knowledge that constituted the bedrock of medical practice. Because of its close identification with myth and superstition, medicine was in the hands of the ancient priesthoods from the beginning. As these early societies became more socially articulated and complex, the priesthood developed into one of the primary social institutions. Its claim to power and status originated in the priests' ability to deal with the unseen and unknown, and because the reasons for illness, disease, and death were unknown, medicine became heavily contaminated with religious explanations for these occurrences. The consequence was that the practice of medicine was controlled by the priesthood and strongly influenced and governed by religious beliefs.

With a few exceptions, notably in Egypt and India, religious beliefs served to hinder the development of empirical medical knowledge among the priest-physicians. The stimulus to producing clinical medical pragmatics was war and the need of the warrior monarchs to preserve their armies from illness, disease, and injury. In almost all cases, clinical medicine grew in response to the needs of the battlefield, and the dominant priest–physician practitioners of religious medicine accorded only secondary social status to the clinicians who practiced it. Perhaps these military medical providers received so little notice because the causes of war injuries were so clearly evident and, thus, required no magical or mystical explanations as other aspects of medicine did. Perhaps it was the press of political reality—that is, the monarchs' need to preserve the army—that forced the priesthoods to relinquish control of the more empirical aspects of medicine while retaining control of the more magical elements. Whatever the reasons, the medical establishments of the ancient world tended to be divided along magical and empirical lines, with clinical practice taking second place.

In those societies where the priesthoods retained effective control of the medical establishment—Egypt, Israel, Persia, and feudal Europe—clinical medical practice either developed more slowly than elsewhere (Egypt), failed to develop at all (Israel), or was almost driven to extinction and uselessness (feudal Europe). In cases where dominant religious control of medical knowledge was combined with a relatively unsophisticated social structure (Germanic barbarians, Persia, Israel, Islam), clinical medicine was almost nonexistent. As a specific application of clinical medicine, military medicine tended to reach its greatest heights in those societies (Rome) that had no strongly established religious priesthoods at all. Even in enlightened Byzantium, the caretaker of the empirical traditions of Greece and Rome, medicine could do no more than survive in cold storage under the religious strictures of the Christian church.

The one example that runs contrary to this trend was the military medicine of the Hindus. The strongly religious origins and nature of Hindu medicine evolved to where religious and empirical treatments for disease, illness, and injury were clinically combined in such a way as to produce the world's first example of holistic medicine in which psychic and physical treatments received equal value. Other than this case, religion and empirical medical pragmatics stood at opposite ends of the spectrum, each fearful of the other's power.

The most effective clinical medicine was practiced in the armies of the ancient world. It was here that physicians, freed from the strictures of religiously derived medical theory and continually faced with the pressing need to aid the wounded, developed the most effective treatment techniques. To the degree that armies trained their own physicians, military surgeons made some of the most important advances in medicine. For example, in an army that wore no helmets, Egyptian military physicians developed treatment techniques for dealing with skull fractures. Sumerian battle surgeons recognized and named the clinical conditions associated with infected wounds. Roman military doctors invented and used the tourniquet and the arterial clamp, and Hindu military doctors contributed greatly to the advancement of battlefield surgery. Military physicians first conceptualized and then introduced field hospitals, ambulance corps, medics, and other means of supporting the medical treatment of the wounded. It is interesting, if frightening, to contemplate in what state medical knowledge might have remained had it not been for the stimulus of war and the contributions of the battle surgeon.

Notes

1. For a fascinating list of the innovations of the Sumerians, see Samuel Noah Kramer, *From the Tablets of Sumer: Twenty-five Firsts in Man's Recorded History* (Indian Hills, CO: Falcon's Wing Press, 1956).
2. Gabriel and Metz, *A History of Military Medicine,* 1:219.

Bibliography

Acharya, A. M. "Military Medicine in Ancient India." *Bulletin of the Indian Institute of History of Medicine* 6 (1971): 50–57.

Ackerknecht, Erwin H. *A Short History of Medicine.* Rev. ed. Baltimore: Johns Hopkins University Press, 1982.

Adamson, P. B. "The Influence of Alexander the Great on the Practice of Medicine." *Episteme* 7, no. 3 (1973): 222–30.

———. "The Military Surgeon: His Place in History." *Journal of the Royal Army Medical Corps* 128, no. 1 (1982): 41–44.

Adcock, F. E. *The Greek and Macedonian Art of War.* Berkeley: University of California Press, 1957.

———. *The Roman Art of War under the Republic.* Cambridge, MA: Harvard University Press, 1940.

Albarracin Teulon, Agustin. "La cirugia Homerica." *Episteme* 5 (1971): 83–97.

Albright, W. F. *The Archaeology of Palestine.* New York: Penguin, 1960.

Aldea, Peter, and William Shaw. "The Evolution of the Surgical Management of Severe Lower Extremity Trauma." *Clinics in Plastic Surgery* 13, no. 4 (October 1986): 549–69.

Alexander, Franz G., and Sheldon T. Selesnick. *The History of Psychiatry: An Evaluation of Psychiatric Thought and Practice from Prehistoric Times to the Present.* New York: Harper & Row, 1966.

Allbutt, Sir T. C. *Greek Medicine in Rome.* London: Macmillan, 1921.

———. *The Historical Relations of Medicine and Surgery to the End of the Sixteenth Century.* London: Macmillan, 1905.

———. *Science and Medieval Thought.* London: C. J. Clay and Sons, 1901.

Alston, Mary Niven. "The Attitude of the Church towards Dissection before 1500." *Bulletin of the History of Medicine* 16, no. 3 (October 1944): 221–38.

Amundsen, Darrel W. "The Forensic Role of Physicians in Ptolemaic and Roman Egypt." *Bulletin of the History of Medicine* 53, no. 3 (Fall 1978): 336–53.

———. "The Liability of the Roman Physician in Roman Law." *International Symposium on Society, Medicine, and Law* (March 1972): 17–31.

———. *Medicine, Society, and Faith in the Ancient and Medieval Worlds.* Baltimore: Johns Hopkins University Press, 1995.

———. "Medieval Canon Law on Medical and Surgical Practice by the Clergy." *Bulletin of the History of Medicine* 52 (1978): 22–44.

———. "Visogothic Medical Legislation." *Bulletin of the History of Medicine* 45 (1971): 553–69.

Anderson, J. K. *Military Theory and Practice in the Age of Xenophon.* Berkeley: University of California Press, 1970.

———. "Wars and Military Science: Greece." In *Civilization of the Ancient Mediterranean: Greece and Rome*, edited by Michael Grant and Rachel Kitzinger. New York: Scribner's, 1988.

Andorlini, Isabella. "L'apporto dei papyri alla conoscenza della scienza medica antica." *Aufstieg und Niedergang der römischen Welt (ANRW)* 2 (1993): 458–562.

Archaeological Survey of Nubia. Bulletins 1–7. Cairo: Ministry of Finance, Survey Department, 1910.

Ardant du Picq, Charles Jean Jacques Joseph. *Battle Studies: Ancient and Modern Battle.* Translated by John N. Greely and Robert C. Cotton. Harrisburg, PA: Military Service Publishing Company, 1947.

Army Veterinary Department. *Animal Management.* London: War Office, 1908.

Arnold, Harry L. "Serpent Emblems in Medicine." *Journal of the Michigan State Medical Society* 36, no. 157 (March 1937): 7–16.

Arrianus (Arrian), Lucius Flavius. *The Campaigns of Alexander.* Translated by Aubrey de Selincourt. London: Penguin, 1958.

"Art of Aswins: Medical Aid on the Battlefield of Ancient India." *Journal of the Indian Medical Association* 13, no. 12 (1943): 850–58.

Asclépiodote, Traité de tactique. Edited by Lucien Poznanski. Paris: Les Belles Lettres, 1992.

Atiyeh, Maurice. "Arab Hospitals in History." *King Faisal Specialist Hospital Medical Journal* 2, no. 2 (1982): 121–26.

Baader, Gerhard. "Early Medieval Latin Adaptations of Byzantine Medicine in Western Europe." *Dumbarton Oaks Papers,* Symposium on Byzantine Medicine 38 (1984): 251–59.

Baker, Raymond W. "History of Egyptian Civilization." In *Encyclopaedia Britannica,* 15th ed. Chicago: Encyclopaedia Britannica, 1985.

Barnett, William S. "Only the Bad Died Young in the Ancient Middle East." *Journal of International Aging and Human Development* 21, no. 2 (1985): 155–60.

Berger, Stephen A., and Stephen C. Edberg. "Infection and Disease in Persons of Leadership." *Reviews of Infectious Diseases* 6, no. 6 (November–December 1984): 802–13.

Berry, Stephan. "Genes of the Phalangites: Bioarchaeology and the Ancient Battlefield." *Ancient Warfare* 4, no. 2 (2010): 46–47.

Bhishagratna, K. K., trans. *Sushruta Samhita.* Calcutta, 1907.

Biggs, Robert. "Medicine in Ancient Mesopotamia." In *A History of Medicine*, edited by A. C. Crombie and M. A. Hoskins, 93–116. Cambridge, MA: Harvard University Press, 1969.

Billings, J. S. "The History and Literature of Surgery." In *System of Surgery*, edited by F. Dennis. Philadelphia: Lea Brothers, 1895.

Birley, E. *Roman Britain and the Roman Army.* Kendal, UK: T. Wilson, 1953.

Black, Jeremy, and Anthony Green. *Gods, Demons, and Symbols of Ancient Mesopotamia: An Illustrated Dictionary.* Austin: University of Texas Press, 1992.

Bliquez, Lawrence T. "Roman Surgical Instruments in the Johns Hopkins University Institute of the History of Medicine." *Bulletin of the History of Medicine* 56 (Summer 1982): 195–217.

———. "Two Lists of Greek Surgical Instruments and the State of Surgery in Byzantine Times." *Dumbarton Oaks Papers,* Symposium on Byzantine Medicine 38 (1984): 187–204.

Bock, Barbara. "On Medicine and Magic in Ancient Mesopotamia." *Journal of Near Eastern Studies* 62, no. 1 (January 2003): 1–16.

Braden, Donald. "The Athenian Casualty Lists." *Classical Quarterly* 63 (1969): 145–59.

Breasted, J. H. *The Edwin Smith Surgical Papyrus.* Chicago: University of Chicago Press, 1930.

Briau, René. *Du service de santé militaire chez les Romains.* Paris: Victor Masson, 1894.

Brothwell, Don, and A. T. Sandison, eds. *Diseases in Antiquity: A Survey of the Diseases, Injuries, and Surgery of Early Populations.* Springfield, IL: Charles C. Thomas, 1967.

Browing, R. "A Further Testimony to Human Dissection in the Byzantine World." *Bulletin of the History of Medicine* 59, no. 4 (Winter 1985): 518–20.

Bullough, Vern L. "Status and Medieval Medicine." *Journal of Health and Human Behavior* 2 (1901): 206–7.

Buringh, P. "Living Conditions in the Lower Mesopotamian Plain in Ancient Times." *Sumer* 13 (1985): 30–46.

Burkill, T. A. "Medicine in Ancient Israel." *Central African Journal of Medicine* 23, no. 7 (July 1977): 153–56.

Burn, A. R. *Persia and the Greeks.* London: Arnold Press, 1962.

Callahan, Dennis J., and Bernard J. Harris. "A Short History of Plaster-of-Paris Cast Immobilization." *Minnesota Medicine* 69 (April 1986).

Callies, Horst. "Zur Stellung der medici im römischen Heer." *MHJ* 3 (1968): 18–27.

Campbell, D. *Arabian Medicine and Its Influence on the Middle Ages.* London: Macmillan, 1926.

Campbell, R. "Assyrian Prescriptions for Diseases of the Head." *American Journal of Semitic Languages* 24 (1907): 1–6.

Casarini, Arturo. "La medicina militare nella leggenda e nella storia." Rome: Collana medico-militare publicata dal Ministero Della Guerre, 1929.

Caspers, Elisabeth. "Sumer, Coastal Arabia, and the Indus Valley in Protoliterate and

Early Dynastic Eras: Supporting Evidence for a Cultural Linkage." *Journal of the Economic and Social History of the Orient* 22, no. 2 (May 1979): 42–49.

Celsus. *De Medicina.* Translated by W. G. Spencer. 3 vols. London: Cambridge University Press, 1961.

Chamberlain, Weston P. "History of Military Medicine and Its Contributions to Science." *Boston Medical and Surgical Journal,* April 1917, 235–49.

Chaplin, Dorothea. *Some Aspects of Hindu Medical Treatment.* London: Luzac, 1930.

Charaka-Samhita. Translated by Avinash Chandra Kaviratna. Calcutta.

Childe, Gordon V. "Horses, Chariots, and Battle Axes." *Antiquity* 15 (1941): 196–99.

Clarke, T. H. M. "Prehistoric Sanitation in Crete." *British Medical Journal* 2 (1903): 597–99.

Coblentz, S. A. *From Arrow to Atom Bomb: The Psychological History of War.* New York: Beechhurst Press, 1953.

Codellas, Pan S. "The Pantocrator: The Imperial Byzantine Medical Center of the 12th Century A.D. in Constantinople." *Bulletin of the History of Medicine* 12 (1942): 392–410.

Cohen-Haft, L. *The Public Physicians of Ancient Greece.* Northampton, MA: Smith College Studies in History, 1956.

Collingwood, R. G., and R. P. Wright. *The Roman Inscriptions of Britain.* Oxford: Clarendon Press, 1965.

Connolly, Peter. *Greece and Rome at War.* Englewood Cliffs, NJ: Prentice-Hall, 1981.

———. *The Greek Armies.* Morristown, NJ: Silver Burdett Company, 1985.

Contenau, Georges. *Everyday Life in Babylon and Assyria.* Translated by K. R. Maxwell-Hyslop and A. R. Maxwell-Hyslop. London: Edward Arnold Publishers, 1954.

———. *La Médicine en Assyrie et en Babylonie.* Paris: Librairie Maloine, 1938.

Cornell, Tim, Boris Rankov, and Philip Sabin. *The Second Punic War: A Reappraisal.* London: Institute of Classical Studies, University of London, 1996.

Corner, G. W. *Anatomical Texts of the Early Middle Ages.* Washington, DC: Carnegie Institution, 1927.

Cottrell, Leonard. *The Warrior Pharaohs.* New York: Putnam, 1969.

Coughlan, H. "The Evolution of the Axe from Prehistoric to Roman Times." *Journal of the Royal Anthropological Society* 73 (1943): 27–56.

Crawford, Harriet. *Sumer and Sumerians.* Cambridge, UK: Cambridge University Press, 1991.

Danforth, John P., and Charles W. Gadd. *A Study of Head and Facial Bone Impact Tolerances.* Warren, MI: General Motors Corporation, 1968.

David, A. Rosalie. *The Ancient Egyptians: Religious Beliefs and Practices.* London: Routledge and Kegan Paul, 1982.

Davies, Roy. "The Medici of the Roman Armed Forces." *Epigraphische Studien* 8 (1969): 83–99.

———. "Medicine in Ancient Rome." *History Today* 21 (1971): 770–78.

———. "The Roman Military Diet." *Britannia* 2 (1971): 122–42.

———. *Service in the Roman Army.* New York: Columbia University Press, 1989.

————. "Some More Military Medici." *Epigraphische Studien* 9 (1972): 1–11.

————. "Some Roman Medicine." *Medical History* 14, no. 1 (January 1970): 101–6.

Davies, T. Witton. "Magic, Divination, and Demonology among the Semites." *American Journal of Semitic Languages and Literature* 14, no. 4 (July 1898): 241–51.

de Filippis Cappai, Chiara. *Medici e medicina in Roma antica*. Turin: Terrenia Stampatori, 1993.

Dehesh, Sindokht. "Pre-Islamic Medicine in Persia." *Middle East Journal of Anaesthesiology* 4, no. 5 (June 1975): 377–82.

Delbrück, Hans. *History of the Art of War within the Framework of Political History.* Translated by Walter J. Renfroe, Jr. 4 vols. Westport, CT: Greenwood, 1975–1985.

Dennis, George T. *Three Byzantine Military Treatises.* Washington, DC: Dumbarton Oaks, Research Library and Collection, 1985.

DePasquale, Anna. "Pharmacognosy: The Oldest Modern Science." *Journal of Ethnopharmacology* 11 (1984): 1–16.

Desai, Prakash N. *Health and Medicine in the Hindu Tradition: Continuity and Cohesion.* New York: Crossroads Press, 1989.

De Vries, Andre, and Abraham Weinberger. "King Asa's Presumed Gout: A 20th Century Discussion of a 9th Century B.C. Biblical Patient." *New York State Journal of Medicine,* February 1975, 452–55.

Diakonoff, M. I. "On the Area and Population of the Sumerian City-State." *Journal of Ancient History* 2 (1950): 77–93.

Dioscorides. *Pedani Dioscordis Anazarbei De Materia Medica.* Edited by Max Wellman. 3 vols. Berlin: Weidmanns, 1907.

Doyle, R. J., and Nancy C. Lee. "Microbes, Warfare, Religion, and Human Institutions." *Canadian Journal of Microbiology* 32, no. 3 (March 1986): 193–203.

Drabkin, I. E. "On Medical Education in Ancient Greece and Rome." *Bulletin of the History of Medicine* 15 (1944): 333–51.

Duffy, Christopher. *The Military Experience in the Age of Reason.* New York: Atheneum, 1988.

Duffy, John. "Byzantine Medicine in the Sixth and Seventh Centuries: Aspects of Teaching and Practice." *Dumbarton Oaks Papers*, Symposium on Byzantine Medicine 38 (1984): 21–27.

Dupuy, Ernest, and Trevor N. Dupuy. *The Encylopedia of Military History from 3500 B.C. to Present.* New York: Harper & Row, 1986.

Dupuy, Trevor N. *The Evolution of Weapons and Warfare.* Indianapolis: Bobbs-Merrill, 1980.

Eadie, J. W. "The Development of Roman Mailed Cavalry." *Journal of Roman Studies* 57 (1967): 161–73.

Edelstein, Ludwig. "Greek Medicine and Its Relation to Religion and Magic." *Bulletin of the Institute of the History of Medicine* 5, no. 3 (March 1937): 201–46.

Eijk, Philip J. van der, H. F. J. Horstmanshoff, and P. H. Schrijvers, eds. *Ancient Medicine in its Socio-Cultural Context: Papers Read at the Congress Held at Leiden University, 13–15 April 1992.* 2 vols. Amsterdam: Editions Rodopi B. V., 1995.

Elgood, Cyril. *Medicine in Persia*. New York: AMS Press, 1978.

Engels, Donald W. *Alexander the Great and the Logistics of the Macedonian Army.* Berkeley: University of California Press, 1978.

Faulkner, R. O. "Egyptian Military Organization." *Journal of Egyptian Archaeology* 39 (1953): 41–47.

Ferngren, Gary B. "Roman Lay Attitudes toward Medical Experimentation." *Bulletin of the History of Medicine* 59 (1985): 495–505.

Ferrill, Arthur. *The Origins of War: From the Stone Age to Alexander the Great.* London: Thames and Hudson, 1985.

Finley, M. I. "The Elderly in Classical Antiquity." *Ageing and Society* 4 (1984): 391–408.

Fishbein, Morris. "The Barber Surgeons and the Liberation of Surgery." *Journal of the International College of Surgeons* 27 (1957): 772–83.

Flemming, Percy. "The Medical Aspects of the Mediæval Monastery in England." *Proceedings of the Royal Society of Medicine* 22, no. 6 (April 1929): 25–36.

Flint, Valerie I. J. *The Rise of Magic in Early Medieval Europe*. Oxford, UK: Clarendon Press, 1991.

Forrest, Richard D. "Development of Wound Therapy from the Dark Ages to the Present." *Journal of the Royal Society of Medicine* 75 (April 1982): 268–73.

Frankel, Walter K. "Medical Symbols and Saints." *Merck Reports* 53, no. 3 (July 1949): 20–25.

Frey, Emile F. "The Caduceus and the Staff of Aesculapius: From Antiquity to the Present." *Texas Reports on Biology and Medicine* 36 (1978): 1–15.

Frölich, Franz Hermann. *Die Militärmedicin Homer's.* Stuttgart: Enke, 1879.

Frost, Harold M. *Orthopaedic Biomechanics*. Springfield, IL: Charles C. Thomas, 1973.

Fulton, John F. "Medicine, Warfare, and History." *Journal of the American Medical Association* 153, no. 5 (October 1953): 427–41.

Gabriel, Richard A. "Amphibious Pharaoh." *Military History,* October–November, 2009, 42–49.

———. *The Culture of War: Invention and Early Development.* Westport, CT: Greenwood, 1990.

———. *Empires at War: A Chronological Encyclopedia.* 3 vols. Westport, CT: Greenwood, 2005.

———. *Gods of Our Fathers: The Memory of Egypt in Judaism and Christianity.* Westport, CT: Greenwood, 2002.

———. *The Great Armies of Antiquity.* Westport, CT: Praeger, 2002.

———. *Hannibal: The Military Biography of Rome's Greatest Enemy.* Washington, DC: Potomac Books, 2010.

———. "The History of Arms." *Italian Encyclopedia of Social Sciences*. Rome: Istituto della Enciclopedia Italiana, 1990.

———. *The Military History of Ancient Israel.* Westport, CT: Praeger, 2003.

———. *Muhammad: Islam's First Great General.* Norman: University of Oklahoma Press, 2007.

————. *No More Heroes: Madness and Psychiatry in War.* New York: Hill and Wang, 1988.

————. *The Painful Field: The Psychiatric Dimension of Modern War.* Westport, CT: Greenwood, 1988.

————. *Philip II of Macedonia: Greater than Alexander.* Washington, DC: Potomac Books, 2010.

————. "The Roman Military Medical Corps." *Military History,* January 2011, 39–43.

————. *Soldiers' Lives through History: Antiquity.* Westport, CT: Greenwood, 2007.

————. *Soviet Military Psychiatry.* Westport, CT: Greenwood, 1986.

————. *Thutmose III: The Military Biography of Egypt's Greatest Warrior King.* Washington, DC: Potomac Books, 2009.

————. "Trajan's Column." *Military History,* September 2010, 43–46.

————. "The Warrior Prophet." *Military History Quarterly* 19, no. 4 (Summer 2007): 6–15.

Gabriel, Richard A., and Karen S. Metz. *From Sumer to Rome: The Military Capabilities of Ancient Armies.* Westport, CT: Greenwood, 1991.

————. *A History of Military Medicine.* 2 vols. Westport, CT: Greenwood, 1992.

Gadd, Charles W., and John P. Danforth. *A Study of Head and Facial Bone Impact Tolerances.* Warren, MI: General Motors Corporation, 1969.

Galen. *Claudii Galeni Opera Omnia.* 22 vols. Edited by C. G. Kuhn. Hildsheim, Germany: Olms Publishers, 1964–1986.

Garrison, Fielding H. "The History of Drainage, Irrigation, Sewage Disposal, and Water Supply." *Bulletin of the New York Academy of Medicine* 5, no. 10 (October 1929): 887–938.

————. *An Introduction to the History of Medicine.* London: W. B. Saunders, 1967.

————. *Notes on the History of Military Medicine.* Washington, DC: Association of Military Surgeons, 1922.

————. "Persian Medicine and Medicine in Persia: A Geomedical Survey." *Bulletin of the History of Medicine* 1, no. 4 (May 1933): 129–53.

————. "The Use of the Caduceus in the Insignia of the Army Medical Officer." *Bulletin of the Military Library Association* 9 (1919): 11–17.

Gilfillan, S. C. "Lead Poisoning and the Fall of Rome." *Journal of Occupational Medicine* 7 (1965): 53–60.

Goffart, Walter. *Barbarians and Romans, A.D. 418–584: The Techniques of Accommodation.* Princeton, NJ: Princeton University Press, 1980.

Goldman, Leon. "Syphilis in the Bible." *Archaeological Dermatology* 103 (May 1971): 535–36.

Gomperz, Heinrich. "Problems and Method of Early Greek Science." *Journal of the History of Ideas* 4, no. 2 (April 1943): 161–76.

Gordon, B. L. "Lay Medicine during the Early Middle Ages." *Journal of the Michigan State Medical Society* 57 (1958): 1006–21.

Gordon, D. S. "Fire and Sword: The Techniques of Destruction." *Antiquity* 27 (1953): 159–62.

————. "Penetrating Head Injuries." *Ulster Medical Journal* 57, no. 1 (April 1988): 1–10.

Gordon, Maurice Bear. *Medicine among the Ancient Hebrews.* Chicago: University of Chicago Press, 1941.

———. "Medicine among the Ancient Hebrews." *Isis* 33, no. 4 (December 1941): 454–85.

Gould, G. M., and W. L. Pyle. "King Arthur's Medicine." *Johns Hopkins Hospital Bulletin* 7 (1897): 239–46.

Grant, Michael. *The Army of the Caesars.* New York: Charles Scribner, 1974.

———. *History of Rome.* New York: Charles Scribner, 1978.

Greenhalgh, P. *Early Greek Warfare: Horsemen and Chariots in the Homeric and Archaic Age.* Cambridge, UK: Cambridge University Press, 1973.

Grivett, Louis Evan, and Rose Marie Pangborn. "Origins of Selected Old Testament Dietary Prohibitions." *Journal of the American Dietetic Association* 65 (December 1974): 634–38.

Grmek, Mirko D. *Diseases in the Ancient Greek World.* Translated by Mireille Muellner and Leonard Muellner. Baltimore: Johns Hopkins University Press, 1989.

Gurdjian, E. Stephen. "The Treatment of Penetrating Wounds of the Brain Sustained in Warfare." *Journal of Neurosurgery* 39 (February 1974): 157–66.

Guterbock, Hans G. "Hittite Medicine." *Bulletin of the History of Medicine* 36 (1962): 109–13.

Haberling, W. "Die Militarlazarette im alten Rom." *Deutsche Militararztliche Zeitschrift* 11 (1909): 441–67.

Hamarneh, Sami. "Development of Hospitals in Islam." *Journal of the History of Medical Allied Sciences* 17, no. 3 (1962): 379–87.

———. "The Physician and the Health Professions in Medieval Islam." *Bulletin of the New York Academy of Medicine* 47, no. 9 (1971): 1088–1112.

———. "Sources and Development of Arabic Medical Therapy and Pharmacology." *Sudhoff's Archive* 54, no. 1 (June 1970): 30–48.

———. "Surgical Development in Medieval Arabic Medicine." *Viewpoint* 5 (1965): 14–18.

Hammond, W. A., ed. *Military Medical and Surgical Essays.* Philadelphia: J. B. Lippincott, 1864.

Hardie, J. B. "Medicine and the Biblical World." *Canadian Medical Association Journal* 94 (January 1966): 31–36.

Hargreaves, Reginald. "Ally of Defeat." *The Practitioner* 202 (May 1960): 713–18.

———. "The Long Road to Military Hygiene." *The Practitioner* 196 (March 1966): 439–47.

Harig, Georg. "Disease, Bible, and Spade." *Biblical Archaeology* 41 (December 1978): 185–86.

———. "Zum Problem 'Krankenhaus' in der Antike." *Klio* 54 (1971): 179–95.

Harrison, R. K. *Healing Herbs of the Bible.* Leiden: E. J. Brill, 1966.

Hartung, Edward F. "Medical Education in the 12th Century." *Medical Life* 41 (1934): 21–26.

Harvey, William. *Exercitatio Anatomica de Motu Cordis et Sanguinis in Animalibus*. Translated by G. Whitteridge. London: Blackwell Scientific Publications, 1976.

Hasel, Gerhard F. "Health and Healing in the Old Testament." *Andrews University Seminary Studies* 21, no. 3 (Autumn 1983): 191–202.

Heager, H. "Army Surgeons in Ancient Greek Warfare." *Journal of Philology* 8 (November 1879): 14–17.

Herodotus. *Herodoti Historiae*. Edited by Carolus Hude. 2 vols. Oxford: Oxford University Press, 1976.

Herzfeld, E. *Zoroaster and His World*. Princeton, NJ: Princeton University Press, 1947.

Herzog, Chaim, and Mordechai Gichon. *Battles of the Bible*. Jerusalem: Steimatzky's Agency Ltd., 1978.

Hignett, C. *Xerxes' Invasion of Greece*. New York: Oxford University Press, 1963.

Hippocratic Corpus. *Oeuvres complètes d'Hippocrate*. Edited by Emile Littré. 10 vols. Paris: Bailliere, 1861.

Historical Statistics of the United States, Colonial Times to 1970. Washington, DC: Department of the Census, 1975.

Hoenig, Leonard J. "Ben Achiya: The First Gastroenterologist in Ancient Israel." *Gastroenterology* 11, no. 1 (1989): 61–63.

Hoffman, Michael A. *Egypt before the Pharoahs*. New York: Knopf, 1979.

Holmes, Bayard, and P. Gad Kitterman. *Medicine in Ancient Egypt: The Hieratic Material*. Cincinnati: Lancet Clinic Press, 1914.

Hooper, David. "Some Persian Drugs." *Bulletin of Miscellaneous Information* 31, no. 6 (1931): 299–344.

Hope, V. M., and E. Marshall, eds. *Death and Disease in the Ancient City*. London: Routledge, 2000.

Hume, Edgar Erskine. "Medical Work of the Knights Hospitallers of St. John in Jerusalem." Paper, New York Academy of Medicine, 1936.

———. *The Military Sanitation of Moses in Light of Modern Knowledge*. Carlisle Barracks, PA: Medical Service Field School, 1940.

Huxley, H. H. "Greek Doctor and Roman Patient." *Greece and Rome* 4, no. 2 (October 1957): 132–38.

Isaac, Eric. "Circumcision as a Covenant Rite." *Anthropos* 59 (1969): 441–44.

Jackson, Ralph. "Roman Doctors and Their Instruments: Recent Research into Ancient Practice." *Journal of Roman Archives* 3 (1990): 1–27.

———. *The Surgeon and the Army*. Norman: University of Oklahoma Press, 1988.

Jacob, Irene, and Walter Jacob, eds. *The Healing Past: Pharmaceuticals in the Biblical and Rabbinic World*. New York: E. J. Brill, 1993.

Jacob, O. "Les cités Grecques et les blessés de guerre." In *Mélanges Gustav Glitz* (Festschrift), II (1932): 461–81.

Jakobovits, Immanuel. "The Dissection of the Dead in Jewish Law: A Comparative and Historical Study." *Tradition* 1, no. 1 (1958): 77–103.

Jarcho, Saul. "Medical and Nonmedical Comments on Cato and Varro with Historical

Observations on the Concept of Infection." *Bulletin of the New York Academy of Medicine* 18 (January 1976): 372–78.

———. "A Roman Experience with Heatstroke in 24 B.C." *Bulletin of the New York Academy of Medicine* 43, no. 8 (August 1967): 767–68.

Joines, Karen Randolph. "The Bronze Serpent in the Israelite Cult." *Journal of Biblical Literature* 87, no. 2 (September 1968): 245–56.

Jones, W. H. S. *Malaria and Greek History.* London: Sherratt and Hughes for the Victoria University of Manchester, 1909.

Josephus, Flavius. *Jewish Antiquities.* Translated by William Whiston. London: Wordsworth Editions, 2006.

———. *The Jewish War.* Translated by G. A. Williamson. London: Penguin, 1984.

Kanner, Leo. "Mistletoe, Magic, and Medicine." *Bulletin of the History of Medicine* 7, no. 8 (October 1939): 875–936.

Kebric, Robert B. "Old Age, the Ancient Military, and Alexander's Army." *The Gerontologist* 28, no. 3 (1988): 298–302.

Kerkhoff, A. H. M. "La médicine dans Homère, une bibliographie." *Janus* 62, nos. 1–3 (1975): 43–49.

Kerstein, Morris, and Roger Hubbard. "Heat-Related Problems in the Desert: The Environment Can Be the Enemy." *Military Medicine* 149 (December 1984): 650–56.

Khadduri, Majid. "Sumerian Civilization." In *Encyclopaedia Britannica,* 15th ed., vol. 21. Chicago: Encyclopaedia Britannica, 1985.

Kinnier Wilson, J. V. "Gleanings from the Iraq Medical Journals." *Journal of Near Eastern Studies* 27, no. 3 (1968): 240–51.

———. "An Introduction to Babylonian Psychiatry." In *Studies in Honor of Benno Landsberger,* 289–98. Chicago: University of Chicago Press, 1965.

———. "Medicine in the Land and Times of the Old Testament." In *Studies in the Period of David and Solomon and Other Essays,* edited by Tomoo Ishida, 337–47. Winona Lake, IN: Eisenbrauns, 1982.

———. "Mental Diseases of Ancient Mesopotamia." In Brothwell and Sandison, *Diseases in Antiquity.*

———. "Two Medical Texts from Nimrud." *Iraq* 18, no. 2 (Autumn 1956): 130–46.

Kirk, N. T. "The Development of Amputation." *Bulletin of the Medical Library Association* 32, no. 2 (April 1944): 132–63.

Kirkup, J. R. "History and Evolution of Surgical Instruments." *Annals of the Royal College of Surgeons in England* 63, no. 4 (1981): 279–85.

Kottek, Samuel S. "The Hospital in Jewish History." *Reviews of Infectious Diseases* 3, no. 4 (July–August 1981): 636–39.

———. *Medicine and Hygiene in the Works of Flavius Josephus.* New York: E. J. Brill, 1994.

Kouretas, D. "The Oracle of Trophonius: A Kind of Shock Treatment Associated with Sensory Deprivation in Ancient Greece." *British Journal of Psychiatry* 113, no. 505 (1979): 1441–46.

Kramer, Samuel Noah. *From the Tablets of Sumer: Twenty-five Firsts in Man's Recorded History.* Indian Hills, CO: Falcon's Wing Press, 1956.

————. "The Oldest Medical Text in Man's Recorded History: A Sumerian Physician's Prescription Book of 4000 Years Ago." *Illustrated London News* 226 (February 26, 1955): 370–71.

————. *The Sumerians: Their History, Culture, and Character.* Chicago: University of Chicago Press, 1963.

Krentz, Peter. "Casualties in Hoplite Battles." *Greek, Roman, and Byzantine Studies* 26, no. 1 (1985): 13–20.

Kudlien, Fridolf. "Early Greek Primitive Medicine." *Clio Medica* 3 (1968): 305–36.

————. "Medical Education in Classical Antiquity." In *The History of Medical Education,* edited by C. D. O'Malley. Berkeley: University of California Press, 1970.

Künzl, Ernst. "Die medizinische Versorgung der römischen Armee zur Zeit des Kaisers Augustus und die Reaktion der Römer auf die Situation bei den Kelten und Germanen." In *Die römische Okkupation nördlich der Aleph zur Zeit des Augustus,* edited by B. Trier, 185–202. Munster, 1991.

Laffont, Robert. *The Ancient Art of Warfare.* 2 vols. New York: Time-Life, 1966.

Lambert, W. G. "A Middle Assyrian Medical Text." *Iraq* 31, no. 1 (Spring 1969): 28–39.

Lawrence, A. W. "Ancient Fortifications." *Journal of Egyptian Archaeology* 51 (1965): 69–94.

Lawrence, Christopher. "The Healing Serpent: The Snake in Medical Iconography." *Ulster Medical Journal* 47, no. 2 (1978): 132–40.

Leibowitz, Joshua O. "Maimonides on Medical Practice." *Bulletin of the History of Medicine* 31, no. 4 (1957): 309–17.

Levey, Martin. *Chemistry and Chemical Technology in Ancient Mesopotamia.* New York: Elsevier, 1959.

————. "Evidences of Ancient Distillation, Sublimation, and Extraction in Mesopotamia." *Centaurus* 4, no. 1 (1955): 23–33.

————. "Some Aspects of the Nomenclature of Arabic Materia Medica." Paper presented at American Association of the History of Medicine, Los Angeles, May 1962.

————. "Some Objective Factors of Babylonian Medicine in Light of New Evidence." *Bulletin of the History of Medicine* 35 (January–February 1961): 61–70.

Levin, S. "Bacteriology in the Bible." *Expository Times* 75 (1964–1965): 154–157.

Levin, Simon S. *Adam's Rib: Essays on Biblical Medicine.* Los Altos, CA: Geron-X Press, 1970.

————. "Job's Syndrome." *Journal of Pediatrics* 76, no. 2 (February 1970): 325–28.

Levy, Reuben. *A Baghdad Chronicle.* Cambridge, UK: Cambridge University Press, 1929.

Lind, Levi Robert. "Popular Knowledge of Anatomy and Medicine in Greece before Hippocrates." *Italian Journal of Archaeology* 83, nos. 1–2 (1978): 33–52.

Lindskog, G. E. "Some Historical Aspects of Thoracic Trauma." *Journal of Thoracic and Cardiovascular Surgery* 42 (1961): 1–11.

Lisowski, F. P. "Prehistoric and Early Historic Trepanation." In Brothwell and Sandison, *Diseases in Antiquity,* 651–72.

Littauer, M. A., and J. H. Crouwel. *Wheeled Vehicles and Ridden Animals in the Ancient Near East.* Leiden: E. J. Brill, 1979.

Littman, R. J., and M. L. Littman. "The Athenian Plague: Smallpox." *Transactions and Proceedings of the American Philological Association* 100 (1969): 261–75.

Liver, J. *The Military History of the Land of Israel in Biblical Times.* Jerusalem: Steinmatzky, 1964.

Lloyd, Seton. *The Archaeology of Mesopotamia: From the Old Stone Age to the Persian Conquest.* London: Thames and Hudson, 1978.

London, P. S. "An Example to Us All: The Military Approach to the Care of the Injured." *Journal of the Royal Army Medical Corps* 134, no. 2 (June 1988): 81–90.

Longrigg, James. *Greek Medicine: From the Heroic to the Hellenistic Age, a Source Book.* New York: Routledge, 1998.

Luckenbill, D. D. *Ancient Records of Assyria and Babylon.* 2 vols. Chicago: University of Chicago Press, 1926.

———. "Assyrian Drugs and Medicine." *American Journal of Semitic Languages and Literatures* 42, no. 2 (January 1926): 138–39.

Macdonell, W. R. "On the Expectation of Life in Ancient Rome, and in the Provinces of Hispania and Lusitania, and Africa." *Biometrika* 9, nos. 3–4 (October 1913): 366–80.

Macht, David I. "A Biblical Adventure in Anatomy." *Bulletin of the History of Medicine* 16 (1944): 169–74.

Majno, Guido. *The Healing Hand: Man and Wound in the Ancient World.* Cambridge, MA: Harvard University Press, 1975.

Manitius, W. "The Army and Military Organization of the Assyrian Kings." *Zeitschrift für Assyriologie* 24 (1910): 90–100.

Marg, Walter. "Kampf und Tod in der Ilias." *WJA* 2 (1976): 7–19.

Marsden, E. W. *Greek and Roman Artillery.* Oxford, UK: Clarendon Press, 1971.

Masterman, E. W. G. "Hygiene and Disease in Palestine in Modern and Biblical Times." *Palestine Exploration Fund Quarterly* 50 (1918): 13–20.

Mathias, Mildred E. "Magic, Myth, and Medicine." *Economic Botany* 48, no. 1 (January–March 1994): 3–7.

Matthew, Christopher. *On the Wings of Eagles: The Reforms of Gaius Marius and the Creation of Rome's First Professional Soldiers.* Newcastle upon Tyne, UK: Cambridge Scholars Publishing, 2010.

———. *A Storm of Spears: A Reappraisal of Hoplite Combat.* London: Pen and Sword, 2010.

Mayer, Claudius. "The Collection of Arabic Medical Literature in the Army Medical Library." *Bulletin of the History of Medicine* 12 (1942): 210–16.

Mazzini, Innocenzo. "La chirurgia celsiana nella storia della chirurgia greco-romana." In *Medecins et medicine dans l'antiquite,* edited by Guy Sabbah, 135–66. Saint-Etienee, 1982.

McCord, Carey P. "Scurvy as an Occupational Disease." *Journal of Occupational Medicine* 13, no. 12 (December 1971): 586–92.

McGrew, Roderick E. *Encyclopedia of Medical History.* With Margaret McGrew. New York: McGraw-Hill, 1985.

McMiken, D. F. "Ancient Origins of Horsemanship." *Equine Veterinary Journal* 22, no. 2 (1990): 73–78.

McPherson, James. *Ordeal by Fire: The Civil War and Reconstruction.* New York: Knopf, 1982.

Mellaart, James. *The Neolithic of the Near East.* New York: Scribner, 1975.

Meyerhoff, Max. "Mediaeval Jewish Physicians in the Near East, from Arabic Sources." *Isis* 28 (May 1938): 440–448.

———. "Sultan Saladin's Physician on the Transmission of Greek Medicine to the Arabs." *Bulletin of the History of Medicine* 18 (1945): 169–78.

Miller, Timothy S. *The Birth of the Hospital in the Byzantine Empire.* Baltimore: Johns Hopkins University Press, 1985.

———. "Byzantine Hospitals." *Dumbarton Oaks Papers*, Symposium on Byzantine Medicine 38 (1984): 53–63.

Milne, J. S. "Galen's Knowledge of Anatomy." *International Medical Congress Proceedings,* sect. 23 (1914): 433–44.

———. *Surgical Instruments in Greek and Roman Times.* London: Clarendon Press, 1907.

Mitchell, Piers D. *Medicine in the Crusades: Warfare, Wounds, and the Medieval Surgeon.* New York: Cambridge University Press, 2004.

Molière, Humbert. "Le service de santé militaire chez les Grecs et les Romains." *Lyon Medical* 58 (1888): 402–8.

Monro, J. K. "The History of Plaster-of-Paris in the Treatment of Fractures." *British Journal of Surgery* 23 (1935): 257–64.

Morcos, S. R., and W. R. Morcos. "Diets in Ancient Egypt." *Journal of Progress in Food and Nutritional Science* 2, no. 10 (1977): 457–71.

Muntner, Z. "Persian Medicine and Its Relation to Jewish and Other Medical Science." *Hebrew Medical Journal* 25 (1952): 197–216.

Neuberger, Max. *History of Medicine.* Translated by E. Playfair. London: Oxford University Press, 1925.

Neufeld, Edward. "Hygiene Conditions in Ancient Israel (Iron Age)." *Journal of the History of Medicine*, October 1970, 414–37.

Neugebauer, O. "The Survival of Babylonian Methods in the Exact Sciences of Antiquity and the Middle Ages." *Proceedings of the American Philosophical Society* 107, no. 6 (December 1963): 528–35.

Newark, Timothy. *The Barbarians: Warriors and Wars of the Dark Ages.* London: Blanford Press, 1985.

Neyrey, Jerome. "Jesus the Devil: Witchcraft Accusations in Matthew." *Abstracts, American Academy of Religion and Society of Biblical Literature,* 1981, 180–92.

Nissen, Hans J. *The Early History of the Ancient Near East, 9000–2000 B.C.* Chicago: University of Chicago Press, 1988.

Nunn, John F. *Ancient Egyptian Medicine.* Norman: University of Oklahoma Press, 1996.

Nutton, Vivian. "Archiatri and the medical profession in antiquity." *Papers of the British School in Rome* 45 (1977): 191–226.

———. "Medicine and the Roman Army: A Further Reconsideration." *Medical History* 13, no. 3 (1969): 260–70.

———. "The Seeds of Disease: An Explanation of Contagion and Infection from the Greeks to the Renaissance." *Medical History* 27 (1983): 1–34.

Oates, J. "The Background and Development of Farming Communities in Mesopotamia and the Zagros." *Proceedings of the Prehistoric Society* 39 (1973): 147–81.

O'Connell, Robert L. *Of Arms and Men: A History of War, Weapons, and Aggression.* New York: Oxford University Press, 1989.

———. "The Roman Killing Machine." *Quarterly Journal of Military History,* Autumn 1988, 30–41.

O'Connor, David. "The Hyksos Period in Egypt." In Oren, *The Hyksos.*

O'Leary, De Lacey. *How Greek Science Passed to the Arabs.* London: Routledge and K. Paul, 1949.

Olmstead, A. T. *The History of Assyria.* Chicago: University of Chicago Press, 1951.

Oman, Charles. *A History of the Art of War in the Middle Ages.* London: Methuen, 1898.

Oppenheim, A. Leo. *Ancient Mesopotamia: Portrait of a Dead Civilization.* Chicago: University of Chicago Press, 1977.

———. "A Caesarian Section in the Second Millennium B.C." *Journal of the History of Medicine and Allied Sciences* 15, no. 3 (1960): 292–99.

———. "Medicine in Babylon and Assyria." *Bulletin of the History of Medicine* 36, no. 2 (March–April 1963): 96–108.

———. "Mesopotamian Medicine." *Bulletin of the History of Medicine* 35, no. 2 (March–April 1962): 97–105.

Oppert, Gustav. *On the Weapons, Army Organisation and Political Maxims of the Ancient Hindus.* Ahmedabad, India: New Order Book Co., 1967.

Oren, Eliezer D., ed. *The Hyksos: New Historical and Archaeological Perspectives.* Philadelphia: University of Pennsylvania Press, 1997.

Oughtred, Orville. "How the Romans Delivered Medical Care along Hadrian's Wall Fortifications." *Michigan Medicine* 79, no. 5 (February 1980): 58–60.

Papageorgiou, M. G. "Incubation as a Form of Psychotherapy in the Care of Patients in Ancient and Modern Greece." *Psychotherapy and Psychosomatics* 26, no. 1 (1975): 35–38.

Parker, H. M. D. "The Legions of Diocletian and Constantine." *Journal of Roman Studies* 23 (1933): 175–89.

"Peep into Medical Care on the Battlefields of India." *Armed Forces Medical Journal* 22, no. 4 (1916): 239–50.

Penn, R. G. "Medical Services of the Roman Army." *Journal of the Royal Army Medical Corps* 110 (1964): 253–58.

———. *Medicine on Ancient Greek and Roman Coins.* London: Seaby, 1994.

Petrov, Boris O. "Study of Ibn Sina's Medical Heritage." *International Congress of the History of Medicine,* Barcelona, 1980, 746–50.

Pfeiffer, Charles F., ed. *The Biblical World: A Dictionary of Biblical Archaeology.* Grand Rapids, MI: Baker Book House, 1966.

Piggott, Stuart. "The Beginnings of Wheeled Transport." *Scientific American* 219, no. 7 (1968): 82–90.

Pilch, John J. "The Health Care System in Matthew: A Social Science Analysis." *Biblical Theology Bulletin* 16, no. 3 (July 1980): 102–6.

Podgorny, George. "Islamic-Persian Medical Education." *North Carolina Medical Journal* 27, no. 3 (1966): 135–40.

Postgate, J. N. "The Assyrian Army at Zamua." *Iraq* 62 (2000): 89–108.

———. *Taxation and Conscription in the Assyrian Empire.* Rome: Biblical Institute Press, 1974.

Pouchelle, Marie-Christine. *The Body and Surgery in the Middle Ages.* Translated by Rosemary Morris. New Brunswick, NJ: Rutgers University Press, 1990.

Preuss, Julius. *Julius Preuss' Biblical and Talmudic Medicine.* Translated by Fred Rosner. New York: Sanhedrin Press, 1978.

The Professional Guide to Disease. Springhouse, PA: Intermed Communications, 1982.

Proskauer, Curt. "A Pictorial History of Dentistry, Part 1—Prehistoric, Egyptian, Assyrian." *TIC Journal* 38, no. 2 (February 1979): 8–11.

Rahman, Abdur, M. A. Alvi, S. A. Khan Ghori, and K. V. Samba Murthy. *Science and Technology in Medieval India: A Bibliography of Source Materials in Sanskrit, Arabic, and Persian.* New Delhi: Indian Natural Sciences Academy, 1982.

Ralston, Bruce. "I Swear by Imhotep the Physician." *New York State Journal of Medicine* 77, no. 13 (November 1977): 2148–52.

Reade, J. E. "The Neo-Assyrian Court and Army: Evidence from the Sculptures." *Iraq* 34, no. 2 (1972): 87–112.

Reiner, E. "Medicine in Ancient Mesopotamia." *Journal of the International College of Surgeons* 41 (1964): 544–50.

Rice, Tamara Talbot. *Everyday Life in Byzantium.* New York: Putnam, 1967.

Richmond, A. "The Roman Army Medical Service." *University of Durham Medical Gazette,* June 1952, 2–6.

Richmond, A., and J. St. Joseph. "On the Legionary Fortress at Inchtuthil." *Journal of Roman Studies* 47 (1957): 198–99.

Riesman, David. *The Story of Medicine in the Middle Ages.* New York: P. B. Hoeber, 1935.

Ritter, Edith. "Magical Expert (=ASIPU) and Physician (=ASU): Notes on Two Complementary Professions in Babylonian Medicine." In *Studies in Honor of Benno Landsberger, Assyriological Studies,* 299–31. Chicago: University of Chicago Press, 1965.

Romano, John. "Temples, Asylums, or Hospitals?" *Journal of the National Association of Private Psychiatric Hospitals* 9, no. 4 (Summer 1978): 5–12.

Rosen, George. *A History of Public Health.* New York: MD Publications, 1958.

Rosen, Z., and J. T. Davidson. "Respiratory Resuscitation in Ancient Hebrew Sources." *Anesthesia and Analgesia* 51, no. 4 (July–August 1972): 498–506.

Rosenthal, Frank. "The Physician in Medieval Muslim Society." *Bulletin of the History of Medicine* 52, no. 4 (Winter 1978): 475–91.

Ross, James A. "Men in Battle: Factors Affecting Their Lives and Well-being." *Journal of the Royal Army Medical Corps* 126, no. 1 (1980): 4–17.

Roux, Georges. *Ancient Iraq.* New York: Penguin, 1986.

Rowe, Norman Lester. "The History of the Treatment of Maxillo-Facial Trauma." *Annals of the Royal College of Surgeons* 49, no. 5 (1971): 329–49.

Sabin, Philip. "The Mechanics of Battle in the Second Punic War." In Cornell, Rankov, and Sabin, *The Second Punic War.*

Saggs, H. W. F. "Assyrian Warfare in the Sargonid Period." *Iraq* 25, part 2 (Autumn 1963): 141–49.

————. *The Greatness That Was Babylon: A Sketch of the Ancient Civilization of the Tigris-Euphrates Valley.* New York: Hawthorn Books, 1962.

————. *The Might That Was Assyria.* London: Sidgwick & Jackson, 1984.

————. "The Nimrud Letters." *Iraq* 36, part 9 (1974): 199–212.

————, W. von Solden, and B. Hrouda. "The Assyrian Army." *Iraq* 25 (1963): 131–66.

Salazar, Christine. "Die Verwundetenfursorge in Heerlen des griechischen Altertums." *AGM* 82, no. 1 (1998): 92–97.

————. *The Treatment of War Wounds in Graeco-Roman Antiquity.* Boston: Brill, 2000.

Salmon, E. T. "The Roman Army and the Disintegration of the Empire." *Proceedings of the Royal Society of Canada* 52 (1958): 43–60.

Sander, Erich. "Zur Rangordnung des römischen Heeres: Der Duplicarius." *Historia* 8, no. 2 (1959): 239–47.

Sarton, George. *Galen of Pergamon.* Lawrence: University of Kansas Press, 1954.

Saxey, Roderick. "A Physician's Reflections on Old Testament Medicine." *Dialogue* 17, no. 3 (Autumn 1984): 122–28.

Scarborough, John. "Early Byzantine Pharmacology." *Dumbarton Oaks Papers*, Symposium on Byzantine Medicine 38 (1984): 213–32.

————, ed. *Folklore and Folk Medicines.* Madison, WI: American Institute of the History of Pharmacy, 1987.

————. "Galen and the Gladiators." *Episteme* 5 (1971): 98–111.

————. "On Medications for Burns in Classic Antiquity." *Clinics in Plastic Surgery* 10, no. 4 (October 1983): 603–10.

————. *Roman Medicine.* London: Thames and Hudson, 1969.

————. "Roman Medicine and the Legions: A Reconsideration." *Medical History* 12, no. 3 (1968): 254–61.

————. "Romans and Physicians." *Classical Journal* 65 (1970): 296–306.

Schoental, R. "A Corner of History: Moses and Mycotoxins." *Preventive Medicine* 9, no. 1 (1980): 159–61.

————. "Mycotoxins and the Bible." *Perspectives in Biology and Medicine* 28, no. 1 (Autumn 1984): 117–20.

Schönberger, H. "The Roman Frontier Army in Germany: An Archaeological Survey." *Journal of Roman Studies* 59, nos. 1–2 (1969): 144–97.

Schulman, Alan R. *Military Rank, Title, and Organization in the Egyptian New Kingdom*. Berlin: Bruno Hessling Verlag, 1964.

Schultz, Rudolf. "Die römische Legionen lazarette in Vetera und andersen Legionslagern." *Bonn Journal* 139 (1934): 54–63.

Scurlock, JoAnn, and Burton R. Andersen, trans. *Diagnoses in Assyrian and Babylonian Medicine: Ancient Sources, Translations, and Modern Medical Analyses*. Urbana: University of Illinois Press, 2005.

Senn, N. "Pompeian Surgery and Surgical Instruments." *The Medical News*, December 28, 1895.

Service, M. W. "A Short History of Early Medical Entomology." *Journal of Medical Entomology* 17, no. 6 (June 1978): 603–26.

Sho, James. *Religion, Mythology, and the Art of War: Comparative Religious Symbolisms of Military Violence*. Westport, CT: Greenwood, 1981.

Sigerist, Henry E. *A History of Medicine*. New York: Oxford University Press, 1961.

———. *A History of Medicine*. Vol. 2, *Early Greek, Hindu and Persian Medicine*. New York: Oxford University Press, 1961.

———. "Materia Medica in the Middle Ages." *Bulletin of the History of Medicine* 7 (1939): 417–27.

———. "The Physician's Profession through the Ages." In *History of Medicine*. New York: MD Publications, 1960.

Simpson, Sir James Y. "Was the Roman Army Provided with Medical Officers?" *Archaeological Essays* 2 (1872): 197–227.

Singer, Charles. *Greek Biology and Greek Medicine*. New York: Oxford University Press, 1922.

———. "Thirteenth Century Miniatures Illustrating Medieval Medical Practice." *Proceedings of the Royal Society of Medicine* 9, no. 35 (1915–1916): 14–29.

Smith, Morton. *Jesus the Magician: Charlatan or Son of God?* Berkeley, CA: Seastone, 1998.

Smith, P. E. L. "Iran, 9000 to 4000 B.C.: The Neolithic." *Expedition* 13 (1971): 3–13.

Spalinger, Anthony. *Aspects of the Military Documents of the Ancient Egyptians*. New Haven, CT: Yale University Press, 1982.

Stannard, Jerry. "Aspects of Byzantine Materia Medica." *Dumbarton Oaks Papers*, Symposium on Byzantine Medicine 38 (1984): 205–11.

Starr, Chester G. *A History of the Ancient World*. New York: Oxford University Press, 1974.

Steinman, Alan. "Adverse Effects of Heat and Cold on Military Operations: History and Current Solutions." *Military Medicine* 152 (August 1987): 382–90.

Steuer, Robert O., and J. B. de C. M. Saunders. *Ancient Egyptian and Indian Medicine: The Relationship of Their Aetiological Concepts of Disease*. Berkeley: University of California Press, 1959.

Sticker, G. *Essays in the History of Medicine*. London: Sudhoff-Festschrift, 1924.

Subbarayappa, B. V. "Medicine and Life Sciences in India." In *Fundamental Indian Ideas of Physics, Chemistry, Life Sciences and Medicine*. Part 2, vol. 4 of *History of*

Science, Philosophy and Culture in Indian Civilization. New Delhi: Munshiram Manoharlal Publishers, 2002.

Surgery of Theodoric (A.D. 1267). Translated by E. Campbell and J. Colton. Vol. 1. New York: Appleton-Century-Crofts, 1955.

Sussmann, Muntner. "The Antiquity of Asaph the Physician and His Editorship of the Earliest Hebrew Book of Medicine." *Bulletin of the History of Medicine* 25, no. 2 (1951): 101–31.

Sykes, Sir Percy. *A History of Persia.* 2 vols. London: Macmillan, 1955.

Tadmor, H. "The Campaigns of Sargon II of Assur." *Journal of Cuneiform Studies* 12 (1958): 22–46.

Taton, René. *History of Science: Ancient and Medieval Science From The Beginning to 1450.* Translated by A. J. Pomerans. New York: 1903.

Temkin, Owsei. "Byzantine Medicine: Tradition and Empiricism." *Dumbarton Oaks Papers* 16 (1962): 95–115.

Thapliyal, U. P. "Military Organization in the Ancient Period." In *Historical Perspectives of Warfare in India: Some Morale and Materiel Determinants,* edited by S. N. Prasad. Vol. 10, part 3. New Delhi: Centre for Studies in Civilizations, 2002.

Thompson, R. Campbell. *Assyrian Medical Texts.* London: John Bale and Sons, 1924.

———. "Assyrian Prescriptions for Diseases of the Head." *American Journal of Semitic Languages and Literatures* 24, no. 1 (October 1907): 323–53.

———. "Assyrian Prescriptions for Treating Bruises and Swellings." *American Journal of Semitic Languages and Literatures* 47, no. 1 (October 1930): 1–25.

Thorwald, J. *Science and Secrets of Early Medicine: Egypt, Mesopotamia, India, China, Mexico, Peru.* London: Thames and Hudson, 1962.

Thucydides. *History of the Peloponnesian War.* Translated by M. I. Finely. London: Penguin, 1972.

Toledo-Pereyra, Luis H. "Galen's Contribution to Surgery." *Journal of the History of Medicine* 28, no. 4 (October 1973): 357–75.

Toy, Sidney. *A History of Fortification from 3000 B.C. to A.D. 1700.* London: Heinemann, 1955.

U.S. Army, Mounted Service School, Fort Riley, KS. *The Army Horse in Accident and Disease.* Washington, DC: U.S. Government Printing Office, 1905.

Van Beek, G. W. "Frankincense and Myrrh." *Biblical Archaeologist* 23 (1960): 70–95.

Vaughn, P. Byron. "Local Cold Injury—Menace to Military Operations: A Review." *Military Medicine* 145, no. 5 (May 1980): 297–308.

Vegetius, Flavius Renatus. *On Roman Military Matters: A 5th Century Training Manual in Organization, Weapons, and Tactics, as Practiced by the Roman Legions.* Translated by John Clarke. London: Red and Black Publishers, 2008.

Vencl, S. "War and Warfare in Archaeology." *Journal of Anthropological Archaeology* 3 (1984): 116–32.

Wagner, Robert, and Benjamin Slivko. "History of Nonpenetrating Chest Trauma and Its Treatment." *Maryland Medical Journal* 37, no. 4 (April 1988): 297–304.

Wangensteen, O. H., J. Smith, and S. D. Wangensteen. "Some Highlights in the History of Amputation Reflecting Lessons in Wound Healing." *Bulletin of the History of Medicine* 41, no. 2 (1967): 97–131.

Watson, G. R. *The Roman Soldier*. Ithaca, NY: Cornell University Press, 1969.

Webster, Graham. *The Roman Army: An Illustrated Study*. Chester, UK: Grosvenor Press, 1956.

———. *The Roman Imperial Army of the First and Second Centuries A.D.* Totowa, NJ: Barnes & Noble, 1985.

Weiss, Gerald N. "The Jews Contribution to Medicine." *Medical Times* 96, no. 8 (August 1968): 791–99.

Wells, Calvin. "Prehistoric and Historical Changes in Nutritional Diseases and Associated Conditions." *Progress in Food and Nutrition Science* 1, no. 11 (1975): 729–79.

Wenke, Robert J. *Patterns in Prehistory: Mankind's First Three Million Years*. New York: Oxford University Press, 1980.

West, Charles G. H. "A Short History of the Management of Penetrating Missile Injuries of the Head." *Surgical Neurology* 16, no. 2 (August 1981): 145–49.

Whipple, A. O. "Role of the Nestorians as the Connecting Link between Greek and Arabic Medicine." *Annals of Medical History* 8 (1936): 313–23.

Wilkins, R. H. "Neurosurgical Classic 17: The Edwin Smith Surgical Papyrus." *Journal of Neurosurgery* 2, no. 14 (1964): 140–44.

Wilmanns, Juliane C. *Die Sanitätdienst im Römischen Reich: Eine sozialgeschichtliche Studie zum römischen Militärsanitätswesen nebst einer Prosopographie des Sanitätspersonals*. Zurich: Medizin der Antike 2, 1995.

Wilson, John A. "Medicine in Ancient Egypt." *Bulletin of the History of Medicine* 36, no. 2 (March–April 1962): 114–23.

———. "A Note on the Edwin Smith Surgical Papyrus." *Journal of Near Eastern Studies* 11, no. 1 (1952): 76–80.

Wilson, Pearl Cleveland. "Battle Scenes in the Iliad." *Classical Journal* 47, no. 7 (1952): 269–74.

Wolff, B. Berthold, and Sarah Langley. "Cultural Factors and the Response to Pain." In *Culture, Disease, and Healing: Studies in Medical Anthropology*, edited by David Landy, 313–19. New York: Macmillan, 1977.

Wood, Percival. *Moses: The Founder of Preventive Medicine*. New York: Macmillan, 1920.

Wood, S. "Homer's Surgeons: Machaon and Podalirius." *Lancet* 1 (1931): 892–95; 947–48.

Wooden, A. C. "Medical Care in Islamic Armies." *International Congress of the History of Medicine* (1980): 694–98.

Yadin, Yigael. *The Art of Warfare in Biblical Lands in Light of Archaeological Study*. Translated by M. Pearlman. 2 vols. New York: McGraw-Hill, 1963.

Yahuda. A. S. "The Osiris Cult and the Designation of Osiris Idols in the Bible." *Journal of Near Eastern Studies* 3, no. 3 (1944): 194–97.

Yates, A. C. "The Knights Hospitallers and the Ambulance Work in War." *Journal of United Services Institute*, 1900, 1099–1138.

Yuval, A. "The Military Medical Service during the Second Punic War According to Livius XXI–XXX." *Koroth* 5, no. 5–6 (1970): 51–58.

Zimmer, H. R. *Hindu Medicine*. Edited by Ludwig Edelstein. Baltimore: Johns Hopkins University Press, 1948.

Zoka, Yaha. *The Imperial Iranian Army from Cyrus to Pahlavi*. Tehran: Ministry of Culture and Arts Press, 1971.

Zun, Ofer. "The Psychohistory of Warfare: The Co-Evolution of Culture, Psyche, and Enemy." *Journal of Peace Research* 24 (1987): 125–34.

Index

About the Author

Richard Gabriel was professor of politics and history and director of advanced courses in the Department of National Security and Strategy at the U.S. Army War College, and has held faculty positions at the University of New Hampshire, University of Massachusetts, and St. Anselm College. He held the Visiting Chair in Ethics at the Marine Corps University, and currently is a distinguished professor in the Department of History and War Studies at the Royal Military College of Canada. Professor Gabriel has also held positions at the Brookings Institution, the U.S. Army Intelligence School, the Center for the Study of Intelligence at the CIA, the Department of Combat Psychiatry at the Walter Reed Army Institute of Research, and the Canadian Forces College in Toronto. Gabriel is the author of forty-six books and more than one hundred articles on various subjects in political science, ancient history, military history, anthropology, psychology, psychiatry, sociology, ethics, philosophy, and the history of theology. His books have been published in German, French, Hebrew, Polish, and Russian. He has delivered over one hundred conference papers in his forty-two-year career. He was awarded an honorary doctorate by the Royal Military College of Canada in 2006. Commissioned a second lieutenant in the U.S. Army in 1964, Gabriel spent twenty years on active and reserve service, retiring at the rank of major. He is married to Susan, is the father of two daughters, and lives in New Hampshire, where he takes great joy in flying his antique open-cockpit Jenny 4D biplane.